SpringerBriefs in Applied Sciences and Technology

Computational Intelligence

Series Editor

Janusz Kacprzyk, Systems Research Institute, Polish Academy of Sciences, Warsaw, Poland

SpringerBriefs in Computational Intelligence are a series of slim high-quality publications encompassing the entire spectrum of Computational Intelligence. Featuring compact volumes of 50 to 125 pages (approximately 20,000–45,000 words), Briefs are shorter than a conventional book but longer than a journal article. Thus Briefs serve as timely, concise tools for students, researchers, and professionals.

More information about this subseries at http://www.springer.com/series/10618

Amit Joshi · Nilanjan Dey · K. C. Santosh
Editors

Intelligent Systems and Methods to Combat Covid-19

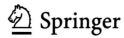 Springer

Editors
Amit Joshi
Global Knowledge Research Foundation
Ahmedabad, Gujarat, India

Nilanjan Dey
Department of Information Technology
Techno International New Town
Kolkata, West Bengal, India

K. C. Santosh
Department of Computer Science
University of South Dakota
Vermillion, SD, USA

ISSN 2191-530X   ISSN 2191-5318   (electronic)
SpringerBriefs in Applied Sciences and Technology
ISSN 2625-3704   ISSN 2625-3712   (electronic)
SpringerBriefs in Computational Intelligence
ISBN 978-981-15-6571-7   ISBN 978-981-15-6572-4   (eBook)
https://doi.org/10.1007/978-981-15-6572-4

This Springer imprint is published by the registered company Springer Nature Singapore Pte Ltd.
The registered company address is: 152 Beach Road, #21-01/04 Gateway East, Singapore 189721,
Singapore

Preface

Since December 2019, the novel coronavirus disease (COVID-19) pandemic (originated from Wuhan, China) has caused serious threats to humanity across the globe. Even though its mortality has not been determined yet, its spreading rate is exponential (dated May 04, 2020).

In this book, several different intelligent systems and methods are proposed to prevent further COVID-19 spreading. The intelligent systems and methods, in this book, include artificial intelligence, machine learning, computer vision, signal processing, pattern recognition, and robotics, just to name a few. To make it clear, the book is not limited to detect/screen COVID-19-positive cases using one type of data, such as radiological image data. They also include how data analytics-based tools can help predict/project further pandemic, where socioeconomic impacts are also taken into account. As COVID-19 has a lot of uncertainties that are primarily due to multiple factors in collecting data, several issues/challenges, such as social distancing (including opportunities), are discussed. As the robustness of AI-driven tools depends on how big the data collection is, we also discuss unavoidable issues in using apps, where data collection, its privacy, and security issues are crucial. To combat COVID-19, not limited to just data analytics-based tools for projection using time series data and pattern analysis tools for unusual pattern discovery (anomaly detection) in image data, AI-enabled robotics and the possible usages are addressed.

In a nutshell, this book primarily aims to provide a variety of approaches for a large audience: Computing and Methodologies, Health Sciences to Business Analytics.

In Chapter "Data Analytics: COVID-19 Prediction Using Multimodal Data", authors address the use of multimodal data for COVID-19 predictions, where data analytics tools are of primary interest. Such predictions will be useful to accommodate future possible threats.

In Chapter "COVID-19 Apps: Privacy and Security Concerns", author addresses the usefulness of apps to track and predict the possible events/threats that come from COVID-19. It considers the use of smartphone-based apps to track peoples' movement, for example. While making such apps available, authors highlight a few but major issues, such as privacy and security at the time they collect data. In brief, the chapter explores different apps that were developed aiming to combat COVID-19 and the related personal data privacy concerns that arise in the post-coronavirus era.

In Chapter "Coronavirus Outbreak: Multi-Objective Prediction and Optimization", authors provide the insight into the mathematical perception about the coronavirus outbreak and analyze them from prediction and optimization points of view. Very specially, constraints, objectives, and measures are identified, and their association and dependencies are analyzed. In their study, authors observed that the coronavirus outbreak is the constrained multi-objective prediction and optimization problem, and it is time-variant.

In Chapter "AI-Enabled Framework to Prevent COVID-19 from Further Spreading", authors discuss the use of AI-enabled (AIE) framework to prevent further COVID-19 spreading. Authors mainly consider AI-enabled framework, where algorithms such as machine learning (ML) and devices such as Global Positioning System (GPS) can be used to design an innovative automation system. Within this context, authors designed an experimental setup, where AIE framework is designed by considering the scenario of urban and rural regions of the state of Haryana, India.

In Chapter "Artificial Intelligence-Enabled Robotic Drones for COVID-19 Outbreak", authors address the use of AI-enabled robotics to prevent further COVID-19 outbreak spreading. Authors consider the use of drones and robots equipped with IoT devices to collect data so that appropriate actions can be made. With IoT, the power of AI and edge computing is considered, where authors explain big data analytics and deployment of suitable tools/techniques across edge and cloud. In brief, the chapter presents how current AI-enabled robotic drone applications and network connectivity are used to improve their performance and increase efficiency in various situations to fight COVID-19. It provides an in-depth review of the literature in addition to possible future research in edge intelligence, AI-enabled robotics, and intelligent networks.

In Chapter "Understanding and Analysis of Enhanced COVID-19 Chest X-Ray Images", authors address the use of radiological image data to check/observe COVID-19 positive cases. In their study, authors consider chest X-ray images. Authors clearly highlight the importance of image enhancement for AI-driven tools.

In Chapter "Deep Learning-Based COVID-19 Diagnosis and Trend Predictions", authors address the use of deep neural networks to predict and diagnose COVID-19 positive cases. In short, the primary motivation is to adopt deep learning (DL) models to check whether it can support clinical decisions by using radiological image data, i.e., computed tomography (CT) scans. Besides, interestingly, authors extend the standard SEIR model, where the parameters are learned from DL model. Such a modified SEIR model can effectively predict the transmission trend of COVID-19 and can be used for short-term trend prediction of the epidemic.

In Chapter "COVID-19: Loose Ends", authors address the possible loose ends due to COVID-19. With limited data, technologies that are built upon artificial intelligence (AI), robotics (R), and IoT (I), i.e., ARI, and their predictions/forecasts could deviate from what they are. Based on the data available, it is possible to have unwanted outcomes. In short, the chapter discusses the role of ARI and loose ends in their implementation, where three major aspects are listed: AI algorithms in analysis and prediction, the use of robotics in control and prevention of the pandemic, and the role of IoT for the patient monitoring system (PMS).

In Chapter "Social Distancing and Artificial Intelligence—Understanding the Duality in the Times of COVID-19", authors discuss the impact of social distancing during COVID-19 and the proper use of AI tools and techniques. This chapter studies the impact of AI-driven tools on a variety of data that are collected when social distancing is considered.

In Chapter "Post-COVID-19 and Business Analytics", considering post COVID-19, authors highlighted the use of AI tools and techniques on a variety of business models. They enlisted a few major global issues that can assist the policymakers to consider developing a business model to bounce back the world economy after this crisis is over. In particular, the chapter enhances the understanding of stakeholders of business about the importance of application of the AI in businesses in a volatile market in post-COVID-19 period.

Ahmedabad, India   Amit Joshi
Kolkata, India   Nilanjan Dey
Vermillion, USA   K. C. Santosh

Contents

About the Editors

Dr. Amit Joshi is currently the Director of Global Knowledge Research Foundation, also an Entrepreneur & Researcher who has completed his Masters and research in the areas of cloud computing and cryptography in medical imaging. Dr. Joshi has an experience of around 10 years in academic and industry in prestigious organizations. Dr. Joshi is an active member of ACM, IEEE, CSI, AMIE, IACSIT, Singapore, IDES, ACEEE, NPA, and many other professional societies. Currently, Dr. Joshi is the International Chair of InterYIT at International Federation of Information Processing (IFIP, Austria). He has presented and published more than 50 papers in national and international journals/conferences of IEEE and ACM. Dr. Joshi has also edited more than 40 books which are published by Springer, ACM, and other reputed publishers. Dr. Joshi has also organized more than 50 national and international conferences and programs in association with ACM, Springer, and IEEE to name a few across different including India, UK, Europe, USA, Canada, Thailand, Egypt, and many more.

Dr. Nilanjan Dey is an Assistant Professor at the Department of Information Technology at Techno International New Town (Formerly known as Techno India College of Technology), Kolkata, India. He is a Visiting Fellow at the University of Reading, UK, and was an honorary Visiting Scientist at Global Biomedical Technologies Inc., CA, USA (2012–2015). He was awarded his Ph.D. from Jadavpur University in 2015. He has authored/edited more than 75 books with Springer, Elsevier, Wiley, and CRC Press and published more than 300 peer-reviewed research papers. He is the Editor-in-Chief of the International Journal of Ambient Computing and Intelligence, IGI Global. He is the Series Co-Editor of Springer Tracts in Nature-Inspired Computing, Springer Nature; Series Co-Editor of Advances in Ubiquitous Sensing Applications for Healthcare, Elsevier; and Series Editor of Computational Intelligence in Engineering Problem Solving and Intelligent Signal Processing and Data Analysis, CRC.

Dr. K. C. Santosh (IEEE Senior Member) is the Chair and Associate Professor of the Department of Computer Science at the University of South Dakota (USD). Before joining USD, Dr. Santosh worked as a Research Fellow at the US National Library of Medicine (NLM), National Institutes of Health (NIH). He worked as a Postdoctoral Research Scientist at the LORIA Research Centre, Universite de Lorraine, in direct collaboration with ITESOFT, France. He also served as a Research Scientist at the INRIA Nancy Grand Est Research Centre, France, where he has received his Ph.D. diploma in Computer Science. Dr. Santosh has published more than 65 peer-reviewed research articles, 100 conference proceedings, and 7 book chapters. He has authored 4 books, and edited 3 books, 11 journal issues, and 4 conference proceedings. He is currently Editor-In-Chief of IJSIP and an Associate Editor for several journals, such as International Journal of Machine Learning and Cybernetics and IEEE Access. He has also chaired more than 10 international conference events. His research projects have been funded by multiple agencies, including the SDCRGP, Department of Education (DOE), and the National Science Foundation (NSF). Dr. Santosh is the proud recipient of the Presidents Research Excellence Award (USD, 2019) and an award from the Department of Health & Human Services (2014).

Data Analytics: COVID-19 Prediction Using Multimodal Data

Parikshit N. Mahalle, Nilesh P. Sable, Namita P. Mahalle, and Gitanjali R. Shinde

Abstract Globally, there is massive uptake and explosion of data, and the challenge is to address issues like scale, pace, velocity, variety, volume, and complexity of this big data. Considering the recent epidemic in China, modeling of COVID-19 epidemic for cumulative number of infected cases using data available in early phase was big challenge. Being COVID-19 pandemic during very short time span, it is very important to analyze the trend of these spread and infected cases. This chapter presents medical perspective of COVID-19 toward epidemiological triad and the study of state of the art. The main aim of this chapter is to present different predictive analytics techniques available for trend analysis, different models and algorithms, and their comparison. Finally, this chapter concludes with the prediction of COVID-19 using Prophet algorithm indicating more faster spread in short term. These predictions will be useful to government and healthcare communities to initiate appropriate measures to control this outbreak in time.

Keywords COVID-19 · Predictive analytics · Machine learning · Prediction · Pandemic

P. N. Mahalle (✉) · G. R. Shinde
Department of Computer Engineering, STES'S Smt. Kashibai Navale College of Engineering, Pune, Maharashtra 411041, India
e-mail: aalborg.pnm@gmail.com

G. R. Shinde
e-mail: gr83gita@gmail.com

N. P. Sable
Department of Computer Engineering, JSPM's Imperial College of Engineering and Research, Wagholi, Pune, Maharashtra 412207, India
e-mail: drsablenilesh@gmail.com

N. P. Mahalle
Pathology Department, Deenanath Mangeshkar Hospital and Research Center, Pune, Maharashtra 411004, India
e-mail: pnmahalle@gmail.com

© The Author(s), under exclusive license to Springer Nature Singapore Pte Ltd. 2020
A. Joshi et al. (eds.), *Intelligent Systems and Methods to Combat Covid-19*,
SpringerBriefs in Computational Intelligence,
https://doi.org/10.1007/978-981-15-6572-4_1

1   Introduction

A novel human corona virus was originated from China on December 2019, causing a severe potentially fatal respiratory syndrome (COVID-19). The symptoms of COVID-19 may or may not be visual in infected individual; hence, spread rate can be faster as individual himself not aware of the infection [1]. Despite the continuous efforts, the virus has managed to spread in most of the territories in the world; World Health Organization (WHO) has announced COVID-19 as pandemic [2, 3]. Countries throughout the world working cooperatively and openly with one another and coming together as a united front in regards of efforts to bring this situation under control using available information and communication technology (ICT). ICT needs to be critically used to bring the situation under control, and predictive analytics can be empowered using ICT services, tools, and applications. ICT can empower epidemiological study to find the determinants, occurrence, and distribution of health and disease in a defined population in terms of COVID-19.

As study [4] shows that 5–80% of people are tested positive for SARS-COV-2 may be asymptomatic. Predictive analytics using ICT plays an important role as some asymptomatic cases will become symptomatic over a period of time. Artificial intelligence (AI) can be beneficial tool to fight against pandemic like COVID-19. AI models can be used for estimating and predicting spread rate; AI was also used in the past pandemics like Zika-virus in 2015. Due to accurate and fast predictions, spread rate can be minimized by taking necessary precautionary action before the time.

In nutshell, taking into consideration the current scenario a sad reality of the COVID-19 pandemic is that many people have been infected. As per the daily situation report of WHO as on April 09, 2020, the COVID-19 transmission scenario reports 1,436,198 confirmed cases with 85,522 deaths globally. The main contribution of this chapter is comparison of various predictive analytics models and algorithms and their applications to appropriate use cases. This study recommends prophet machine learning algorithm for prediction due to various reasons which are discussed in Sect. 4 of this chapter. Another contribution of this study is to present various avenues to initiate high-quality research in biomedical science along with integrative approach of predictive analytics and mathematical modeling to control outbreak of any pandemic. In the view of above-mentioned-related issues, we should also promote ecumenical and interfaith collaboration and peaceful coexistence during the COVID-19 pandemic.

The main objectives of this chapter are as follows:

1. To understand medical perspective of COVID-19 toward epidemiological triad;
2. To analyze state of the art for different approaches and models used for forecasting and prediction;
3. To understand various predictive analytics models and algorithm as well as their comparison with respect to the use cases;
4. To study the performance of Prophet Algorithm for the prediction of COVID-19.

The remainder of this chapter is organized as below. Section 2 presents medical perspective of COVID-19 in terms of its origin, most infected underline age group, and transmission. Section 3 discusses the analysis of different studies available in the literature for predicting COVID-19. Section 4 presents various predictive analytics models, algorithms, and their comparison. Finally, Sect. 5 concludes the chapter with future outlook.

2 Medical Perspectives

The emergence of SARS-CoV-2 is confirmed from Wuhan's Huanan Seafood market, China, but specific animal source still remains uncertain. There is uncertainty regarding origin of SARS-CoV-2 [5]. The situation with SARS-CoV-2 is developing faster with the numbers of infected cases and death is increasing exponentially. The unprecedented control measures taken have been effective in preventing spreading of SARS-CoV-2. Still, there is continued rise in number of cases with infection of SARS-CoV-2. Hence, it is essential to identify that the increase is due to infected cases before lockdown, due to community transmission; hospital acquired infection or spread within family. This should be determined experimentally, which may help in revealing the actual numbers of infected patients and asymptomatic carriers.

Many studies have confirmed transmission among human of SARS-CoV-2 [6, 7], but mechanism of transmission and pathogenesis in spreading in humans remains to be fully explored? During transmission from human to human, whether the pathogenicity of this virus is decreased with the increase in rate of transmission? If the transmission of this virus is declined, the outbreak may eventually end. Nevertheless, if there is continuous and effective transmission, SARS-CoV-2 will develop into an additional human coronavirus which is community acquired. It is difficult to recognize and take further actions in patient with undefined and mild symptoms. Studying a group of asymptomatic infected cases, and following them for their clinical presentation, titers of antibody and viral loads, will help in understanding about the number of subjects have symptoms later, whether viral shedding is actually less robust and how frequently asymptomatic carriers can transmit virus further. A study reported that asymptomatic infection is high (15.8%) in children under 10 years [8].

COVID-19 can be spread through respiratory droplets or due to close contact with the infected patients. SARS-CoV-2 was isolated from fecal samples of infected patients, which support the significance of feco-oral route in the transmission of SARS-CoV-2, but a WHO-China joint commission report has denied this route of transmission [9]. However, the likelihood of transmission of SARS-CoV-2 through human waste, contaminated water, aerosols, and air conditioners cannot be underestimated; this may have happened in case of Diamond Princess cruise ship, where there was widespread COVID-19 infection [10]. Still, to confirm the role of feco-oral transmission of SARS-CoV-2, further studies will be required. Severe cases caused by the infection of SARS-CoV-2 may develop neurological, respiratory, gastrointestinal, and hepatic complications leading to mortality. Many studies have reported low sense of smell and taste as a manifestation of COVID-19 [11], but whether this is a unique feature of COVID-19 is uncertain. Till date, we do not have definite antiviral drug or vaccine for SARS-CoV-2. However, screening of new drug molecules may prove beneficial in treating COVID-19, which will have therapeutic effect.

Globally, there has been lot of progress in monitoring and control of disease spread. It is evident that there are lot of uncertainties and questions regarding transmission mechanism, asymptomatic or subclinical patient's virus shedding, origin of virus, virus pathogenesis, treatment, symptoms, etc. This highlights the need of integrative approach of predictive analytics and mathematical modeling with biological science, which may help government to take appropriate measures and method for future preparedness in fighting against this outbreak. In spite of rapid progression in research toward this outbreak, most of the studies are unable to suggest and guide effective measures to control this current situation. However, more high-quality research in biomedical science along with predictive analytics and mathematical modeling is warranted to manage public health crisis in short and long terms.

3 Related Works

As per the Italy official release, there are total 27,980 infected cases and 2158 deaths of people who were positive of COVID-19 [12]. Due to rapid spread of COVID-19, in short time many studies have been carried out for prediction of trend and its impact. This section briefs about all such recent studies which are essentially related to predictive analytics. Giordano et al. [12] propose epidemic prediction model that compares infected density and the level of symptoms. Authors have proposed a SIDARTHE Model which helps to redefine reproduction number, and simulation results also show that the proposed model gives accurate results after comparing the findings with real data on the COVID-19 epidemic in Italy. Bannister-Tyrrell et al. [13] presented an interesting study to establish the correlation of temperature and evidence of COVID-19 in Europe. Authors claim that the seasonal variation essentially in the temperature greatly impacts the spread of COVID-19. Study states that higher average temperature is potential candidate to limit the spread of COVID-19. Russo et al. [14] presented a mechanism to find the first day of infections and predictions of COVID-19 in Italy. Depending upon proposed work, authors are able to estimate that the actual count of exposed cases of COVID-19. Volpert et al. [15] nicely presented the effect of quarantine model on the spread of coronavirus infection using data analytics. The main aim of this work is to present the assessment of placed quarantine mechanism using mathematical modeling.

Weber et al. [16] presented the trend analysis of COVID-19 pandemic in China using globally accepted SIR model in this study. The dataset used in this study is taken from Johns Hopkins University site for analysis, and it is found that epidemic was contained in China. The basic aim of the study presented by Zhang et al. [17] is to provide control measures to be considered internationally for global control of this pandemic. The time frame of dataset is from 3 to 10 February, 2020, and authors presented a time series model to predict number of infected cases and the turning point where the spread is at peak. Feasibility analysis of controlling COVID-19 spread by isolating infected cases and quarantine is presented by Hellewell et al. [18]. The proposed probabilistic model presented in this study considered varied scenarios like initial infections, basic reoccur number, and probability of contacts traced and rate of clinical infections. The results show that, in epidemic situation, isolation of infected people and contact tracing is not sufficient to minimize the rate of spread. Modeling of COVID-19 epidemic in China for cumulative number of infected cases using data available in early phase based on differential equation is presented by Liu et al. [19]. Simulation results show that if the restrictions would have been applied one week before, then there would have been significant reduction in the number of infected cases.

Various ML models are discussed in the literature however for better accuracy deep learning models can be used for better predictions [20–22]. Furthermore, predictions can be more accurate using active learning models in this multitudinal and multi-modal data used for predictions instead of single type of data [23]. In addition to this, early forecasting of COVID-19 from small dataset is presented by Fong et al. [24]. Fong et al. [25] have also proposed to use Composite Monte-Carlo simulation forecasting method for helping government to initiate critical actions and decisions to control spread of novel coronavirus. Experimental results using deep learning-based composite Monte-Carlo with fuzzy rule induction show that decision makers are benefited more in the form of better fitted Monte-Carlo outputs.

All the studies discussed above are centric toward prediction and forecasting of COVID-19 based on short-term data available on this pandemic. Literature shows that various mathematical and stochastic theory-based approaches are used for estimation and prediction of spread rate of COVID-19. Most of the studies are giving expected predictions. There are so many predictive analytics models, such as Susceptible-Infection-Recovered (SIR) [26] and Hospital Impact Model for Epidemics (CHIME) [27] which has been working from decades. The SIR models work best in the case where data is not dynamic. In COVID-19, there is frequent change in data; hence, learning model can be suitable for analysis of pandemic data like COVID-19. Prediction of number of hospitals and facilities, i.e., hospital beds and ventilators, is also equally important. In the view of this, predictive healthcare team developed COVID-19 CHIME model at Penn Medicine. These predictions can help hospitals to be prepared for worst-case scenarios.

4 Predictive Analytics

Predictive analytics is specialized branch of data analytics for making better predictions using past data and using analysis techniques which include statistical and learning methods. Discovery of patterns in input data and anticipating what is likely to happen is the main objective of predictive analytics. Statistical analysis, predictive modeling, and machine learning are three main pillars of predictive analytics. The main capabilities of predictive analytics are *statistical analysis, predictive modeling, linear regression, and logistic model.*

Selection of appropriate predictive model and algorithm decide how efficiently we can make the better insights and useful decisions. Use case like hospital interested in prediction of number of patients likely to be admitted in intensive care unit in next seven days and prediction of fraud transaction for online banking provider might require different predictive analytics model than for predicting defaulter applicant for loan provider and predicting number of COVID-19 infected patient in next 10 days. Selection of appropriate predictive model is based on what predictive question would you like to address and how optimization can be carried out using predictive algorithms. The major pillars of predictive analytics are listed below:

1. Predictive Analytics Models;
2. Predictive Analytics Algorithms.

4.1 Predictive Analytics Models

Classification models are best for decision problems where the answer is merely Yes or No. This model classifies data into multiple categories using past data, and the prediction of fraud transaction for online banking provider will come into this model. *Clustering model* arranges data into multiple logical groups based on some common attributes. An interesting use case for this model might be grouping of students into different logical buckets based on marks, city they come from in order to decide the distribution of amount of effort for improving performance. *Forecast model* is another most popular predictive model and mainly applied to the use case where past numerical data is available to predict the value performance metrics or new value using learning from past data. As stated earlier, forecasting number of COVID-19 infected patient in next 10 days will fit into this model. When dataset contains inconsistent data records, *outlier models* are most useful as these models can identify these inconsistent entries. Finding strange records in insurance claim can be solved by this model. *Time series model* are used for short-term predictions using data points collected from the past in time domain (i.e., based on time as input parameter). Collecting short-term data from China epidemic and predicting the same for India can be solved using these models.

4.2 Predictive Analytics Algorithms

Predictive analytics algorithms are either based on machine learning or deep learning. Machine learning algorithms are used when there is a need of classification or clustering for prediction, decision, or analysis. These algorithms are more suitable for structured data and can be linear or nonlinear in nature. Deep learning algorithms are subset of machine learning algorithms and more useful when there is a need of identification or to recognize something. These algorithms are more useful to bigger data like audio, video, and images where machine learning algorithms start underperforming. The predictive analytics is mainly driven by learning techniques, and there are wide ranges of applications for disease prediction in healthcare community [28, 29]. *Random forest* algorithm is based on decision trees and used for both classification and regression purposes. This algorithm is more suitable for big data and uses bagging to avoid the errors. This model can address over fitting more effectively. *Gradient boosted model* is ensemble model of decision tress and used for classification. This model uses incremental model by building one tree at each time by correcting errors made by previously trained tree. In contrast, in random forest there is no relation among trees. *K-means* algorithm works on unlabeled data and places new incoming data into logical groups based on some common feature. Consider the COVID-19 example where clusters are formed of various patients based on some severity of infection. K-mean model is useful to put new incoming patient into appropriate cluster. This method is extremely useful in this growing pandemic of COVID-19 due to large number of cases. Prediction of mortality and spread rate plays very important role in pandemic disease like COVID-19, as based on this prediction precautionary measures can be taken by public, government, and heathcare systems. We have used FBProphet [30] algorithm for training the model and predicting number of infected cases in next three months. We agree that there are many machine learning algorithms present in the literature. However, this study recommends Prophet Algorithm for better prediction because it is mainly an opensource algorithm giving more accurate prediction. As we are aware that in sudden pandemic likes COVID-19, adequate data is not available due to various reasons like duration and lack of required parameters for better prediction, prophet algorithm enables better forecast and does not require dataset training in time series methods. The key features of this algorithm are it works more accurate for time series data and mainly used for prediction and capacity planning. Dataset can be referred from widely accepted sources like John Hopkins University and WHO. In this study, the dataset is referred from Kaggle where the statistics for this COVID-19 pandemic is given in the form of features like state/province, country, latitude, longitude, date, confirmed infected, deaths, and recovered. There are eight fields in the dataset and another feature of Prophet is it does not require splitting of dataset wherein for fitting it takes whole dataset for accurate results. Figures 1 and 2 show the short-term prediction of number of infected cases.

Figures 1 and 2 show the prediction of spread of COVID-19. The numbers of confirmed cases of COVID-19 within respective duration are presented in the graph, X-axis presents the duration and Y-axis shows the number of COVID-19 confirmed cases. ML model is trained for prediction based on the worldwide dataset retrieved from Github. Predictions are shown in Fig. 1 and it shows that the confirmed COVID-19 infected cases would be 1.6 million and 2.3 million by the end of May and June, respectively, and hence can be concluded that with increasing duration spread of COVID-19 increasing and government should initiate appropriate control measures in time to regulate this pandemic.

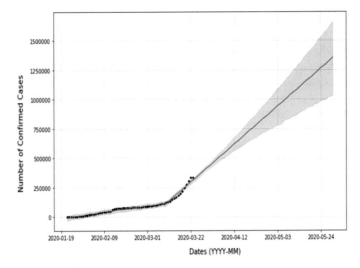

Fig. 1 Prediction of confirmed cases till end of May

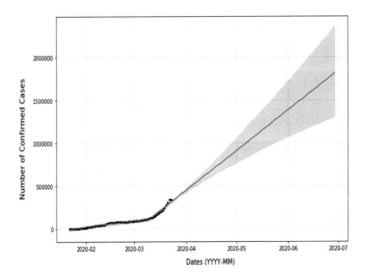

Fig. 2 Prediction of confirmed cases till end of June

5 Conclusion

Due to pandemic of Coronavirus and COVID-19, all countries are looking toward mitigation plan to control the spread with the help of some modeling techniques. This research work aims to understand the complete medical perspective of this COVID-19 pandemic and how predictive analytics will empower the predictions. Analysis of various predictive analytics methods available in the literature is presented in this chapter. We have also discussed and presented the comparative analysis of various predictive analytics models and algorithm by suggesting more appropriate use cases for application. Out study indicates that there is a need of thorough assessment of these predictive analytics algorithm based on the type of question to be answered. Application of prophet predictive analytics algorithm on Kaggle dataset, its predictions are also presented in this chapter. Simulation result of this model shows that the confirmed COVID-19 infected cases would be 1.6 million and 2.3 million by the end of May and June, respectively. We hope that these predictions will be also helpful to pharmaceutical companies to manufacture drugs in faster rate.

References

1. The Novel Corona Virus Pneumonia Emergency Response Epidemiology Team. (2020). The epidemiological characteristics of an outbreak of 2019 novel corona virus diseases (COVID-19)—China, 2020. *China CDC Weekly, 2,* 113–122.
2. WHO. (2020). *Novel corona virus (2019-nCoV) situation report—39.* Cited March 2020. Available from: https://www.who.int/docs/default-source/coronaviruse/situationreports/20200228-sitrep-39-covid-9.pdf.
3. WHO. (2020). *Novel corona virus (2019-nCoV) situation report—52.* Cited March 2020. Available from: https://www.who.int/docs/default-source/coronaviruse/situation-reports/20200312-sitrep-52-covid-19.pdf.
4. *The center of evidence-based medicine develops, promotes and disseminates better evidence for healthcare CEBM-University of OXFORD report.* (2020). Cited April 6, 2020. https://www.cebm.net/covid-19/covid-19-what-proportion-are-asymptomatic/.
5. Singhal, T. (2020). A review of coronavirus disease-2019 (COVID-19). *Indian Journal of Pediatrics, 87*(4), 281–286.
6. Rothe, C., Schunk, M., Sothmann, P., Bretzel, G., Froeschl, G., Wallrauch, C., et al. (2020). Transmission of 2019-nCoV infection from an asymptomatic contact in Germany. *New England Journal of Medicine, 382*(10), 970–971.
7. Chan, J. F. W., Yuan, S., Kok, K. H., To, K. K. W., Chu, H., Yang, J., et al. (2020). A familial cluster of pneumonia associated with the 2019 novel coronavirus indicating person-to-person transmission: A study of a family cluster. *Lancet, 395*(10223), 514–523.
8. Xiaoxia, L., Liqiong, Z., Hui, D., Jingjing, Z., Yuan, L., Jingyu, Q., et al. (2020). SARS-CoV-2 infection in children. *New England Journal of Medicine.* https://doi.org/10.1056/NEJMc2005073.
9. https://www.who.int/docs/default-source/coronaviruse/who-china-joint-mission-on-covid-19-final-report.pdf.
10. Moriarty, L. F., Plucinski, M. M., Marston, B. J., Kurbatova, E. V., Knust, B., Murray, E. L., et al. (2020). Public health responses to COVID-19 outbreaks on cruise ships-worldwide. *MMWR Morbidity and Mortality Weekly Report, 69,* 347–352.
11. Russell, B., Moss, C., Rigg, A., Hopkins, C., Papa, S., & Van Hemelrijck, M. (2020). Anosmia and ageusia are emerging as symptoms in patients with COVID-19: What does the current evidence say? *Ecancer Medical Science, 14,* ed98.
12. Giordano, G., Blanchini, F., Bruno, R., Colaneri, P., Di Filippo, A., Di Matteo, A., & Colaneri, M. (2020). A SIDARTHE model of COVID-19 epidemic in Italy. arXiv preprint arXiv:2003.09861.
13. Bannister-Tyrrell, M., Meyer, A., Faverjon, C., & Cameron, A. (2020). Preliminary evidence that higher temperatures are associated with lower incidence of COVID-19, for cases reported globally up to 29th February 2020. *medRxiv.*

14. Russo, L., Anastassopoulou, C., Tsakris, A., Bifulco, G. N., Campana, E. F., Toraldo, G., & Siettos, C. (2020). Tracing DAY-ZERO and forecasting the fade out of the COVID-19 outbreak in Lombardy, Italy: A compartmental modelling and numerical optimization approach. *medRxiv.*
15. Volpert, V., Banerjee, M., & Petrovskii, S. (2020). On a quarantine model of coronavirus infection and data analysis. *Mathematical Modelling of Natural Phenomena, 15,* 24.
16. Weber, A., Ianelli, F., & Goncalves, S. (2020). Trend analysis of the COVID-19 pandemic in China and the rest of the world. arXiv preprint arXiv:2003.09032.
17. Zhang, F., Zhang, J., Cao, M., & Hui, C. (2020). A simple ecological model captures the transmission pattern of the coronavirus COVID-19 outbreak in China. *medRxiv.*
18. Hellewell, J., Abbott, S., Gimma, A., Bosse, N. I., Jarvis, C. I., Russell, T. W., & Flasche, S. (2020). Feasibility of controlling COVID-19 outbreaks by isolation of cases and contacts. *The Lancet Global Health.*
19. Liu, Z., Magal, P., Seydi, O., & Webb, G. (2020). Predicting the cumulative number of cases for the COVID-19 epidemic in China from early data. arXiv preprint arXiv:2002.12298.
20. Mukherjee, H., Ghosh, S., Dhar, A., Obaidullah, S. M., Santosh, K. C., & Roy, K. (2020). Shallow convolutional neural network for COVID-19 outbreak screening using chest X-rays. https://doi.org/10.36227/techrxiv.12156522.v1.
21. Rajinikanth, V., Dey, N., Raj, A. N. J., Hassanien, A. E., Santosh, K. C., & Raja, N. (2020). Harmony-search and Otsu based system for coronavirus disease (COVID-19) detection using lung CT scan images. arXiv preprint arXiv:2004.03431.
22. Das, D., Santosh, K. C., & Pal, U. (2020). Truncated inception net: COVID-19 outbreak screening using chest X-rays. https://doi.org/10.21203/rs.3.rs-20795/v1.
23. Santosh, K. C. (2020). AI-driven tools for coronavirus outbreak: Need of active learning and cross-population train/test models on multitudinal/multimodal data. *Journal of Medical Systems, 44,* 93. https://doi.org/10.1007/s10916-020-01562-1.
24. Fong, S. J., Li, G., Dey, N., Crespo, R. G., & Herrera-Viedma, E. (2020). Finding an accurate early forecasting model from small dataset: A case of 2019-nCoV novel coronavirus outbreak. arXiv preprint arXiv:2003.10776.
25. Fong, S. J., Li, G., Dey, N., Crespo, R. G., & Herrera-Viedma, E. (2020). Composite Monte Carlo decision making under high uncertainty of novel coronavirus epidemic using hybridized deep learning and fuzzy rule induction. *Applied Soft Computing,* 106282.
26. Teles, P. (2020). Predicting the evolution of SARS-COVID-2 in Portugal using an adapted SIR model previously used in South Korea for the MERS outbreak. arXiv preprint arXiv:2003.10047.
27. http://predictivehealthcare.pennmedicine.org/2020/03/14/accouncing-chime.html.
28. Chen, M., Hao, Y., Hwang, K., Wang, L., & Wang, L. (2017). Disease prediction by machine learning over big data from healthcare communities. *IEEE Access, 5,* 8869–8879.
29. Shinde, G. R., Kalamkar, A. B., Mahalle, P. N., Dey, N., Chaki, J., & Hassanien, A. E. (2020). Forecasting models for coronavirus (COVID-19): A survey of the state-of-the-art. *TechRxiv.* Preprint. https://doi.org/10.36227/techrxiv.12101547.v1.
30. https://facebook.github.io/prophet/docs/quick_start.html.

COVID-19 Apps: Privacy and Security Concerns

Surekha Borra

Abstract Today, with the rapid spread of COVID-19, many governments and start-ups are coming forward to develop smartphone apps that trace where we all are, whom we met and for how long, with a goal of interrupting new chains by informing potentially exposed people. These new platforms make use of anonymous use of Bluetooth technology and GPS, enabled either on smartphones or armbands in order to prepare maps corresponding to quarantine monitoring, contact tracing, movement tracking, social distancing and density reports. With different apps for different countries, one thing most of the apps facilitate is tracking. To save lives during an extraordinary crisis, many governments are willing to overlook privacy implications. Keeping in view that the sensitive data being collected is not exclusive to public health organizations and governments, this chapter explores different apps that were developed aiming to combat COVID-19, and the related personal data privacy concerns that arise in the post-coronavirus era.

Keywords Apps · Bluetooth · COVID-19 · GPS · Privacy · Security

1 Introduction

While the researchers around the world are busy developing COVID-19 related AI-driven tools [1, 2], forecasting methods [3–5], screening [6] and image-assisted decision support systems [7], COVID-19 mobile apps are being developed for a variety of reasons, ranging from quarantine monitoring, contact tracing, movement tracking, social distancing and density reports. All these mobile apps with or without the consent of the user collect user personal information, including location histories and stores the data on the third-party servers, which might lead to serious cyberthreats and associated fears. Hence, reporting the available apps and analysing the side effects including security and privacy concerns is the need of the hour.

S. Borra (✉)
Department of Electronics and Communication Engineering, K.S. Institute of Technology, Bengaluru, Karnataka, India
e-mail: borrasurekha@gmail.com

© The Author(s), under exclusive license to Springer Nature Singapore Pte Ltd. 2020   11
A. Joshi et al. (eds.), *Intelligent Systems and Methods to Combat Covid-19*,
SpringerBriefs in Computational Intelligence,
https://doi.org/10.1007/978-981-15-6572-4_2

While the privacy compromises have prevented more open take-up of such technologies, China used phone tracking for contact tracing successfully apart from voluntary registrations. China made it mandatory for its citizens to install apps on their mobiles, to monitor their movements, and to give instructions [8]. Tools [9] that can detect if someone is not wearing a mask are also in use. These tools can even recognize individuals from just their eyes when wearing masks. China also used drones to monitor sections of the population [10].

Singapore's Trace Together app [11] shares 'proximity information' to Ministry of Health when a user device with the app installed is in the Bluetooth range of a carrier device via Bluetooth, for follow-up actions. Quarantine breaches are monitored by real-time tracking the carriers in Israel using 'anti-terror' technology. Some governments are using GPS phone tracking, Bluetooth technology and credit card records, to track carriers' movements. While location tracking information from mobile companies is being collected by Austria, Germany and Italy, countries like Hong Kong, Singapore, Berlin, South Korea, Australia and Taiwan are using location monitoring systems to map the COVID-19 carriers. To fight the spread of COVID-19, the UK planned to use the databases of mobile network trade association, the GSMA. The Pan-European Privacy-Preserving Proximity Tracing (PEPP-PT) [12], developed by European Union, tracks virus spread by tracking the smartphones. Google and Facebook have recently collaborated with the USA in collecting and monitoring the location history based on smartphone apps.

2 COVID-19 Apps

The conventional way of quarantine monitoring and contract tracing is by humans, which is very much time-consuming and resource intensive. Usage of personal digital devices, installation of software apps, aggregation of Bluetooth, GPS and mobile signals is must in the current scenario. All these technologies assist the authorities in updating the real-time data automatically in a central server at a fast rate, at different scales. The data includes new COVID-19 cases, proximity contacts, social distancing and quarantine status along with the location histories. A variety of apps based on different technologies were developed with respect to COVID-19 in a span of just 4 months by different government authorities, private companies and researchers, some of which are listed in Tables 1 and 2.

The social distance enforcing apps warns the people if they get too close to others or if they spend too much time outside or away from their homes, during the lockdown. The quarantine apps are mandated by the governments like India, Poland, Taiwan. These ask for sharing the GPS location and selfies, to ensure those quarantined at home are not breaking the rules. Switching off their phone or venturing to leave their houses triggers the alert system, police visits, further calls and messages are sent to the concerned person to ascertain their whereabouts. To trace the movements of quarantined and infected people, their contacts and to score the likelihood of infections, the authorities need to know where they had been and who else had

Table 1 COVID-19 apps

App category	Name of the app
Information	Coronavírus—SUS, Pakistan's National Action Plan for COVID-19, TGN Emergències, Atman, iVH HIT, Coronavirus Bolivia, Hamro Swasthya, Apple COVID-19, COVID-19!, Coronavirus Australia
Self-testing or self-assessment of symptoms	Coronavírus—SUS, MySejahtera, Atman, COVID-19 Armenia, Apple COVID-19, Coronavirus Australia, STOP COVID19 CAT
Share experiences of the patients	CoronaReport—COVID-19 reports for social science
Registering health data and follow up	Coronavirus UY, MySejahtera, Kenya COVID-19 Tracker, Karantinas, GVA Coronavirus, HEALTHLYNKED COVID-19 Tracker, PatientSphere for COVID19
COVID-19 test result	ALHOSN UAE
Monitor symptoms and health information	HSE COVID-19, PatientSphere for COVID19, STOP COVID19 CAT
Quarantine	BeAware Bahrain, Kenya COVID-19 Tracker, Karantinas, StayHome App, HSE COVID-19
Contact tracing	BeAware Bahrain, Kenya COVID-19 Tracker, TraceCovid, TraceTogether

been there. Many countries are leveraging cell phone location data from cell phone towers, marketing-style databases, Google, Apple and Facebook Apps to track the spread of the virus.

3 Advantages and Concerns of COVID-19 Apps

With an end goal of reducing the spread of COVID-19, mass information collection strategies are as of now being put to utilize. Conducting interviews with patients in which they detail where they had been and with whom they met in the weeks going before they were tested positive is complex and time taking task, for the governments in this crucial time. Some countries have published comprehensive digital maps and lists of confirmed cases, their movements, and their travel history, by means of personal interviews with patients and surveillance videos. Some governments [13] have published the pre-quarantine movements of people well before they were diagnosed with the virus, gender, age, occupation, address, and where they travelled recently including restaurants, gyms and hospitals [14]. Most of the countries are actively tracking population movements by the CCTV footage, credit card records, cell phone signals and mobile location data to help combat coronavirus. The advantages of such technologies are listed below:

Table 2 COVID-19 apps developed in India

App category	Name of the app
Information	Jaano (service providers for daily needs), GoK Direct—Kerala
Quarantine	COVID-19 Quarantine Monitor Tamil Nadu, MahaKavach, GCC—Corona Monitoring, UP Self-Quarantine App, Corona Mukt Himachal, Quarantine Watch, COPE Odisha, COVID-19 West Bengal Government, SMC COVID-19 Tracker, CoBuddy—Covid19 Tool, Covid Locator, COVID CARE
F/B to administration	Jaano, COVID19 Feedback (f/b on treatment), CoBuddy—Covid19 Tool
Request for COVID-19 test	Niramaya
Call support	COVA Punjab
Reporting symptoms	GCC—Corona Monitoring, Uttarakhand CV 19 Tracking System
Self-testing or self-assessment of symptoms	Aarogya Setu, Kavach, Niramaya, COVA Punjab, Test Yourself Goa, GCC—Corona Monitoring, Test Yourself Puducherry
Contact tracing	Aarogya Setu, Tracetogether, SMC COVID-19 Tracker
Tracking (Geofencing) (GPS)	MahaKavach, CoBuddy—Covid19 Tool, Covid Locator, COVID CARE, Corona Watch (14 days of movement history)
Lockdown pass	KSP Clear Pass Checker, CG Covid-19 ePass

- Eases countrywide lockdowns.
- Speeds up the preventive actions.
- Limits the spread of the virus.
- Manages and tracks virus carriers in a quick way.
- Tracks those at a risk of infection effectively.
- Works automatically and accurately.
- Populates the anonymized map data.
- Enables better management of the evolving situation.
- Enforces government directives with less manpower.
- Estimates asymptomatic carriers' population.
- Helps in identifying where to target critical medical resources.
- Enables researchers and scientists to learn how long the virus survives on a surface.
- Communicates information to the citizens at fast rate.

Apps like Google collect data from those who have turned their GPS ON. While some mobile networks do not give options to the users for their consent to collect their location data, most of the apps ask user permission to track their location history. Some sneaky apps track the locations without the knowledge. Therefore, though the smartphone surveillance might seem like a good solution to tracking the COVID-19 spread, it is far from guaranteed to work and have many data protection and privacy issues and concerns [15–18], some of which are listed below:

- Enable unwanted corporate or government surveillance.
- Apps that collect locations feed this data to marketing companies and are paid to do so.
- Some apps use the information to serve the user more relevant advertisements and content.
- Data more often serves private profit such as advertising.
- Inherent loss of privacy, highly invasive.
- Location tracking apps reveal sensitive information about everything from political dissent to journalists' sources to extramarital affairs.
- Sacrifice of freedom still causes anxiety, despite the clear public interest.
- May sometimes do more harm than good.
- Apps might sometimes sow unnecessary alarm or confusion.
- Possibility of privacy threats from contacts, snoopers and the authorities.
- Announcing the infected people identities stirs up public shaming and rumour-mongering.
- Incorrect information might encourage risky behaviour leads to false sense of security.
- Apps might only provide a very crude picture of the spread.
- It may be challenging to get people install such apps and report their status.
- Once the privacy back door opens, there are chances that it remains permanent.
- Fine-grained location tracking is complex.
- Accuracy may often be less precise.
- Complex database systems involving tagging and monitoring citizens.

4 Discussions and Recommendations

Smartphone apps that model and monitor the spread of diseases based on Bluetooth and other wireless technology were first developed by Jon Crowcroft and Eiko Yoneki at Cambridge University in 2011 [19]. Fluphone [20] asks the people to report the flu-like symptoms, for monitoring the person who got sick, and to let to know who had contacted that person. However, because only 1% of people used that app, tracking and reporting the transmissions was not as expected. With the current COVID-apps and technologies, the concerns are:

- How to reduce trade-offs among the speed of implementation, effectiveness and privacy.
- How well such a system would work and how is it being utilized.
- Whether such systems to be developed and deployed country by country or agree a cross-border solution.
- Whether the apps better deal with this kind of situation next time around.

- Whether more than half the population would trade personal privacy to avoid further lockdowns.

Though there are several implications of utilizing location histories data, here are some recommendations for the authorities and the app developers:

- Governments should ensure trust and privacy principles.
- Keep location data private.
- Avoid surveillance.
- Encryption of information can be done before saving and publication.
- Government should take measures to explain to the citizens, how the apps work, what it gathers, for how long, when it is disposed and for what purpose data is utilized.
- Apps should opt-in and should not last beyond a time of crisis.
- No data records should link back to an individual.
- Any personal data should not leave a device.
- Data itself, though, must be uniquely identifiable.

5 Conclusions

Though the Google's mobility reports and mobile networks data sources are available, these are not used for contact tracing until recently. With the occurrence of new COVID-19 cases developing continuously, the government authorities started harnessing apps and the cell phone location data bases, for monitoring isolation, social distancing and behavioural changes in the war against the spread of the new coronavirus. However, unless majority of population uses the app, the tracking and reporting of the transmissions will not be successful. Practicing digital distancing, restricting the access permissions to apps, confirming if the app is by legitimate developer and downloading the app from trusted mobile app stores can assist in dealing with potential security issues that may arise in future.

References

1. Santosh, K., Das, D., & Pal, U. (2020). Truncated inception net: COVID-19 outbreak screening using chest X-rays.
2. Santosh, K. C. (2020). AI-driven tools for coronavirus outbreak: Need of active learning and cross-population train/test models on multitudinal/multimodal data. *Journal of Medical Systems, 44*(5), 1–5.
3. Fong, S. J., Li, G., Dey, N., Crespo, R. G., & Herrera-Viedma, E. (2020). Finding an accurate early forecasting model from small dataset: A case of 2019-nCoV novel coronavirus outbreak. arXiv preprint arXiv:2003.10776.
4. Fong, S. J., Li, G., Dey, N., Crespo, R. G., & Herrera-Viedma, E. (2020). Composite Monte Carlo decision making under high uncertainty of novel coronavirus epidemic using hybridized deep learning and fuzzy rule induction. *Applied Soft Computing,* 106282.

5. Mahalle, P., Kalamkar, A. B., Dey, N., Chaki, J., & Shinde, G. R. (2020). Forecasting models for coronavirus (COVID-19): A survey of the state-of-the-art.

6. Mukherjee, H., Ghosh, S., Dhar, A., Obaidullah, S., Santosh, K. C., & Roy, K. (2020). Shallow convolutional neural network for COVID-19 outbreak screening using chest X-rays.

7. Rajinikanth, V., Dey, N., Raj, A. N. J., Hassanien, A. E., Santosh, K. C., & Raja, N. (2020). Harmony-search and Otsu based system for coronavirus disease (COVID-19) detection using lung CT scan images. arXiv preprint arXiv:2004.03431.

8. https://www.nytimes.com/2020/03/01/business/china-coronavirus-surveillance.html.

9. https://www.bbc.com/news/technology-51717164.

10. https://www.forbes.com/sites/zakdoffman/2020/03/05/meet-the-coronavirus-spy-drones-that-make-sure-you-stay-home/#1319d4ee1669.

11. Help speed up contact tracing with TraceTogether. (2020, March). *Singapore Government Blog.* [Online]. Available: https://www.gov.sg/article/help-speed-up-contact-tracing-with-tracetogether.

12. PEPP-PT. https://www.pepp-pt.org.

13. http://ncov.mohw.go.kr/en/.

14. Kim, M. J., & Denyer, S. (2020, March). A travel log of the times in South Korea: Mapping the movements of coronavirus carriers. *The Washington Post.* [Online]. Available: https://www.washingtonpost.com/world/asiapacific/coronavirus-south-koreatracking-apps/2020/03/13/2bed568e-5fac-11eaac50-18701e14e06dstory.html.

15. Cho, H., Ippolito, D., & Yu, Y. W. (2020). Contact tracing mobile apps for COVID-19: Privacy considerations and related trade-offs. arXiv preprint arXiv:2003.11511.

16. Berke, A., Bakker, M., Vepakomma, P., Raskar, R., Larson, K., & Pentland, A. (2020). Assessing disease exposure risk with location histories and protecting privacy: A cryptographic approach in response to a global pandemic. arXiv preprint arXiv:2003.14412.

17. Demirag, D., & Ayday, E. (2020). Tracking and controlling the spread of a virus in a privacy-preserving way. arXiv preprint arXiv:2003.13073.

18. Bell, J., Butler, D., Hicks, C., & Crowcroft, J. (2020). TraceSecure: Towards privacy preserving contact tracing. arXiv preprint arXiv:2004.04059.

19. https://www.wired.com/story/phones-track-spread-covid19-good-idea/.

20. https://www.cl.cam.ac.uk/research/srg/netos/projects/archive/fluphone/.

Coronavirus Outbreak: Multi-Objective Prediction and Optimization

Nileshsingh V. Thakur

Abstract Coronavirus disease-19 (COVID-19) is the name given by World Health Organization (WHO) and the cause of this pandemic is severe acute respiratory syndrome-related coronavirus (SARS-CoV-2). This pandemic was started in China and later got spread throughout the world. As of now, it has affected around 213 countries, areas or territories and the world has eyes on it. This chapter provides the insight on mathematical perception about the coronavirus outbreak and is analyzed from prediction and optimization point of view. Constraints, objectives and measures are identified and their association and dependencies are analyzed from mathematical point of view. Four levels and weighting factors are used for the identified constraints. Presented mathematical formulation can evaluate the count of positive cases, mortality, recovery cases, transmission rate and prediction of peak time period. It is observed that the coronavirus outbreak is the constrained multi-objective prediction and optimization problem and also it is time variant.

Keywords COVID-19 · Constrained optimization · Multi-objective prediction · Multi-objective optimization · Mathematical problem

1 Introduction

World Health Organization (WHO) named the present outbreak of a coronavirus-associated acute respiratory disease as coronavirus disease-19 (COVID-19) [1]. The Coronaviridae Study Group (CSG) of the International Committee on Taxonomy of Viruses (ICTV) has classified this virus and tentatively named 2019-nCoV, within the Coronaviridae [2]. This virus has been recognized as severe acute respiratory syndrome coronaviruses (SARS-CoVs) of the species and designated as severe acute respiratory syndrome-related coronavirus (SARS-CoV-2) by CSG. It is reported that the virus might be bat origin [4]. The genetic features and some clinical findings

N. V. Thakur (✉)
Computer Science and Engineering, Prof Ram Meghe College of Engineering and Management, Badnera, India
e-mail: thakurnisvis@rediffmail.com

© The Author(s), under exclusive license to Springer Nature Singapore Pte Ltd. 2020   19
A. Joshi et al. (eds.), *Intelligent Systems and Methods to Combat Covid-19*,
SpringerBriefs in Computational Intelligence,
https://doi.org/10.1007/978-981-15-6572-4_3

of the infection have been reported recently [5–7]. Spread at international level via commercial air travel had been assessed [8].

Uniqueness of COVID-19 can be described by three characteristics—(1) Time delay between real cases and daily reported cases, due to two week incubation period [9], (2) Epidemic trend depends on the available medical resources, preventive and corrective measures and the efficiency of confirmation of positive cases, (3) Quarantine measures are implemented by most of the countries to hold no risk of contagion. Due to the outbreak and control-related distinctiveness of COVID-19 from existing contagious diseases, the existing epidemic models cannot be purposeful to portray the observed data directly. So, it is difficult to describe COVID-19 with Susceptible-Infectious-Recovered (SIR), Susceptible-Exposed-Infectious-Recovered (SEIR), etc. epidemic models [10, 11].

Recently, various research works are reported to detection and prediction of COVID-19 [12–17]. In [12], the authors have proposed the Truncated Inception Net deep learning model which is based on convolutional neural network. The authors have carried out the experimentation on six data sets which are composed of chest X-rays images. In [13], the authors have demonstrated the use of X-rays images for the mass screening to find the COVID-19 positive cases through the light-weight CNN-based shallow architecture which works with less parameters. In [14], authors have used CT scan images to locate the infected region and infection level of severity in the lungs. They have employed the use of Harmony-Search-Optimization and Otsu thresholding for the image enhancement.

The importance of artificial intelligence-driven tools for the prediction of spread rate of COVID-19 is elaborated in [15]. The author has mentioned about the need of cross-population models which should be based on active learning and it should employ the multitudinal and multimodal data. In [16], the authors have proposed the methodology based on polynomial neural network with corrective feedback for the prediction of spread of COVID-19. This methodology is designed with the collection of five optimized forecasting models. The use of deterministic and non-deterministic input data for the prediction of epidemic spread through the stochastic model based on Monte-Carlo model with the use of deep learning network and fuzzy rule induction is described in [17].

As COVID-19 is distinct from the existing contagious diseases, it is difficult to describe coronavirus outbreak by using SIR and SEIR epidemic models. Hence, there is a need of mathematical analysis of coronavirus outbreak with additional parameters. This chapter proposes the mathematical formulation which is based on the preventive measures, corrective measures and identified constraints. This mathematical formulation can evaluate-positive cases count (P), mortality count due to coronavirus (M), transmission rate of coronavirus (T), coronavirus recovery cases count (R) and prediction of peak time period (PP). Four levels and weighting factor is considered for constraint parameters. This chapter describes the coronavirus outbreak as the constrained multi-objective prediction and optimization problem. Relevant mathematical analysis and scope of utilizing artificial intelligence and data science are discussed.

Remaining part of this chapter is organized as follows: Symptoms, prevention and impingement related to coronavirus are briefly described in Sect. 2. Constraints, objectives and measures are identified in view of mathematical perception which is discussed in Sect. 3. Discussion on constrained multi-objective prediction and optimization is provided in Sect. 4. Section 5 elaborates the general idea to use the artificial intelligence and data science followed by conclusion in Sect. 6.

2   Coronavirus: Symptoms, Prevention, Impingement

In general, this virus affects different people in different ways. It is observed that the symptoms are mild to moderate and most of the infected people recover without any special treatment. Coronavirus symptoms and prevention measures are suggested by WHO [1].

Common symptoms include—fever, tiredness and dry cough. Other symptoms include—shortness of breath, aches and pains, sore throat and rare symptoms include diarrhea, nausea or a runny nose. It is intolerant in people who have underlying medical conditions and those over 60 years old, due to a higher risk of developing severe disease and death.

General preventive measures are—*Hand wash*—Wash hands on regular basis with soap and water, or clean with alcohol-based hand rub; *Keep away*—Maintain at least 1 meter distance from coughing or sneezing fellow; *Avoid face touch*—Evade face touching; *Face mask*—Use mask to cover the face which will help to cover mouth and nose when coughing or sneezing; *Avoid outing*—Stay home if not well; *Lungs caring*—Avoid smoking and other activities that weaken the lungs; and *Distancing*—Staying away from large groups of people.

2.1   *Impingement*

On December 31, 2019, the WHO China Country Office was informed of cases of pneumonia unknown etiology (unknown cause) detected in Wuhan City, Hubei Province of China. Till January 3, 2020, a total of 44 case-patients with pneumonia of unknown etiology were reported to WHO by the national authorities in China. The Chinese authorities identified a new type of coronavirus, which was isolated on 7 January 2020. On 13 January 2020, the Ministry of Public Health, Thailand reported the first imported case of lab-confirmed novel coronavirus (2019-nCoV) from Wuhan, Hubei Province, China. Spread of this virus is reported at Japan and Republic of Korea, also. Patient cases in Thailand, Japan and Republic of Korea were exported from Wuhan City, China [1].

As of now, COVID-19 grabbed the whole world which includes 213 countries, areas or territories with 1848439 confirmed cases and 117217 confirmed deaths [18]. The first case in India was reported on 30 January 2020. Since then, to 14 April 2020,

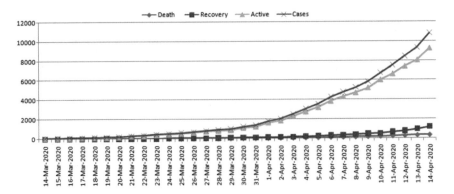

Fig. 1 Statistics of COVID-19 cases in India from March 14 to April 14, 2020

10815 confirmed cases, 1190 recovered cases, 9272 active cases and 353 confirmed deaths are reported [19]. Figure 1 shows the statistics of COVID-19 cases in India from 14 March 2020 to 14 April 2020.

3 Coronavirus Outbreak—Mathematical Perceptions

Due to non-availability of proper medical treatment, coronavirus eruption becomes a tedious task for the government and medical practitioners. Engineering academicians and researchers may contribute to this pandemic by providing mathematical analysis and formulation for the avoidance, prediction, and minimization of spread of COVID-19. Apart from the medical treatment, some typical measures, namely—lockdown, social distancing, home quarantine, isolation, etc. are already adopted, prominently, by China and India. Prominent and concrete mathematical solution have not yet arrived which may perfectly predict and optimize this pandemic. To explore the role of mathematics, some basic mathematical formulation is required.

3.1 Constraints

The aim of any government or healthcare unit of any country is to minimize the impact of COVID-19 pandemic. This impact may be related to the parameters, namely— count of coronavirus positive cases, count of mortality due to coronavirus, social and economical disruption, and mental stress, etc. One has to minimize all these parameters, but, with the existing constraints and some other imposed constraints due to the developed panic of COVID-19. As no drug exists to overcome the COVID-19 and it is a contagious disease, some other measures have to be considered and implemented to avoid the spread of this pandemic. As the incubation period of

Table 1 Constraint parameters with their levels and weight factor

Constraint parameters	Level (weight factor λ)			
Demographic trend (DT)	Kid (10)	Young (10)	Middle (10)	Old (10)
Gravity of existing disease (GD)	Poor (5)	Average (8)	Moderate (9)	Critical (10)
Population count (PC)	Low (5)	Average (8)	Moderate (9)	High (10)
Density of population (DP)	Low (5)	Average (8)	Moderate (9)	High (10)
Living style (LS)	Poor (5)	Average (8)	Moderate (9)	High (10)
Mental stress (MS)	Low (5)	Average (8)	Moderate (9)	High (10)
People connectivity (CO)	Low (5)	Average (8)	Moderate (9)	High (10)
Stage of spread (SS)	Onset (5)	Local (8)	Community (9)	Peak (10)

this disease is of 14 days, it is difficult to guess or predict the number of affected cases. Identified constraint parameters with their levels and weight factor are given in Table 1. To predict and optimize the coronavirus outbreak, existing and imposed constraints have to be considered.

Weight factor (λ) value range is from 5 to 10. COVID-19 is a contagious disease and no drug is available, the probability of becoming coronavirus affected is 0.5 and as the highest weight factor is 10, therefore, the lowest weight factor is considered as 5. Different variants of combinations of these constraints can be used for the mathematical formulation. These constraints weight factor may vary with respect to the locality.

3.2 Objectives and Measures Adopted

Currently, sole aim in COVID-19 pandemic is to have minimum number of coronavirus positive cases. Objectives are identified from mathematical analysis point of view and are divided into two categories—*Minimization* of-coronavirus positive cases count (P), mortality count due to coronavirus (M), transmission rate of coronavirus (T), social and economical disruption (S), and *Maximization* of—coronavirus recovery cases count (R). These objectives have to be optimized to conquer coronavirus effect. Apart from this, another objective is-prediction of peak time period (PP), *i.e.,* the prediction of spread of COVID-19 with the imposition of identified constraints and accordingly proper preventive and corrective measures should be implemented. Therefore, from mathematical point of view, coronavirus outbreak is the multi-objective prediction and optimization problem with imposed constraints.

Following measures are adopted in China and India to minimize the panic of coronavirus outbreak. These measures are divided into two categories—*Preventive measures* (θ) include—personal care (PR), social distancing (SD), lockdown (LD), and house-to-house inspection (HH), and *Corrective measures* (η) include—home quarantine (HQ), institutional quarantine (IQ), medical treatment (MT).

4 Constrained Multi-Objective Prediction and Optimization

The coronavirus outbreak appeared to be nonlinear in nature and time variant. To do the prediction and optimization, bottom-up approach has to be incorporated, i.e., specific to general. Therefore, local prediction and local optimization have to be carried out first to find the global prediction and global optimization. The complete geographic region has to be divided into different sub-regions and then the local evaluation should be carried out. The process of evaluation of proposed mathematical formulation is shown in Fig. 2 where E-Evaluation, P-Prediction and O-Optimization.

With reference to Table 1, total 4^8 constraints can be formulated. Preventive measures adopted affect few of the identified constraints, for example, personal care—affects the constraint GD, LS, MS, CO and social distancing, lockdown, house-to-house inspection—affects the constraint MS, CO. Corrective measures adopted affect few of the identified constraints, for example, home quarantine, institutional quarantine and medical treatment—affects the constraint GD, LS, MS and CO. Other constraints DT, PC, DP and SS remain as it is. Presented mathematical analysis is related to the local evaluation. We can apply it to any local region of the country. Every local region mostly consists of all the types of level for the constraint DT. If so, then based on the percentage evaluation of level, the weight factor value is applicable. Main objectives of this mathematical analysis are—P, M, T, S and R. Out of these, presently, we are considering only P, M, T, R and excluding S as it involves many uncontrolled parameters. P, M, and T are related to the minimization and R is related to the maximization. Identified objectives are associated with other objectives and measures. Identified constraints DT, GD, PC, DP, LS, MS, CO and SS are directly or indirectly associated with P, M, T and R. Objective association with other objectives, measures and constraint parameters is given in Table 2. Associated objectives, measures and constraints sequence is based on relevance, more relevant appears first.

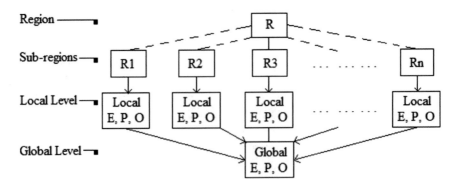

Fig. 2 Process of evaluation of proposed mathematical formulation

Table 2 Objective association—objectives, measures and constraint parameters

Objectives—association with other objectives, preventive measure (θ) and corrective measure (η)	Type	Association with constraints	
		Direct (φ)	Indirect (ϕ)
Positive cases (P)-T and PR, SD, LD, HH, HQ, IQ	Minimization	CO, SS	DP, PC, GD, DT, LS, MS
Mortality (M)-P and MT, HQ, IQ	Minimization	CO, GD, DT, SS, MS	DP, PC, LS
Transmission rate (T)-PR, SD, LD, HH, HQ, IQ	Minimization	SS, CO, DP, PC, LS	GD, DT, MS
Recovery (R)-P, M and MT	Maximization	CO, SS	DP, PC, GD, DT, LS, MS
Prediction (PP)-P, M, T, R and PR, SD, LD, HH, HQ, IQ	Depends on P, M, T, R	All constraints	All constraints

All the computations have to be performed with respect to the time t. Preventive measure (θ) and corrective measure (η) values are in percentage. T, α, β can be evaluated by using moving average of previous days data or cumulative data. Equation 1 through Eq. 8 can be used for the computations. All relevant objective functions, that is, minimization of P, M, T and Maximization of R are subject to the constraints and adopted measures.

$$P_{(t)} = T_{(t)} \cdot P_{(t-1)}, \quad M_{(t)} = \alpha_{(t)} \cdot M_{(t-1)}, \quad R_{(t)} = \beta_{(t)} \cdot R_{(t-1)} \tag{1}$$

$$P_{(t+1)} = \left[\frac{T_{(t)} + T_{(t+1)}}{2} + \frac{1}{10 \cdot n} \sum_{i=1, \, i \in \varphi}^{n=2} \lambda_i + \frac{1}{10 \cdot m} \sum_{j=1, \, j \in \phi}^{m=6} \lambda_j \right.$$
$$\left. - \sum_{k=1, \, k \in \theta}^{k=4} \frac{\theta_k}{100 \cdot k} - \sum_{l=1, \, l \in \eta}^{l=2} \frac{\eta_l}{100 \cdot l} \right] P_{(t)} \tag{2}$$

$$M_{(t+1)} = \left[\frac{\alpha_{(t)} + \alpha_{(t+1)}}{2} + \frac{1}{10 \cdot n} \sum_{i=1, \, i \in \varphi}^{n=5} \lambda_i \right.$$
$$\left. + \frac{1}{10 \cdot m} \sum_{j=1, \, j \in \phi}^{m=3} \lambda_j - \sum_{l=1, \, l \in \eta}^{l=3} \frac{\eta_l}{100 \cdot l} \right] M_{(t)} \tag{3}$$

$$T_{(t+1)} = \left[\frac{1}{10 \cdot n} \sum_{i=1,\, i \in \varphi}^{n=5} \lambda_i + \frac{1}{10 \cdot m} \sum_{j=1,\, j \in \phi}^{m=3} \lambda_j \right.$$
$$\left. - \sum_{k=1,\, k \in \theta}^{k=4} \frac{\theta_k}{100 \cdot k} - \sum_{l=1,\, l \in \eta}^{l=2} \frac{\eta_l}{100 \cdot l} \right] \tag{4}$$

$$\alpha_{(t+1)} = \left[\frac{1}{10 \cdot n} \sum_{i=1,\, i \in \varphi}^{n=5} \lambda_i + \frac{1}{10 \cdot m} \sum_{j=1,\, j \in \phi}^{m=3} \lambda_j - \sum_{l=1,\, l \in \eta}^{l=3} \frac{\eta_l}{100 \cdot l} \right] \tag{5}$$

$$R_{(t+1)} = \left[\frac{\beta_{(t)} + \beta_{(t+1)}}{2} + \frac{1}{10 \cdot n} \sum_{i=1,\, i \in \varphi}^{n=2} \lambda_i + \frac{1}{10 \cdot m} \sum_{j=1,\, j \in \phi}^{m=6} \lambda_j - \sum_{l=1,\, l \in \eta} \frac{\eta_l}{100} \right] R_{(t)} \tag{6}$$

$$\beta_{(t+1)} = \left[\frac{1}{10 \cdot n} \sum_{i=1,\, i \in \varphi}^{n=2} \lambda_i + \frac{1}{10 \cdot m} \sum_{j=1,\, j \in \phi}^{m=6} \lambda_j - \sum_{l=1,\, l \in \eta} \frac{\eta_l}{100} \right] \tag{7}$$

$$PP_{(t+n)} = \left[T_{(t+1)} \cdot P_{(t+1)} + \alpha_{(t+1)} \cdot M_{(t+1)} + \beta_{(t+1)} \cdot R_{(t+1)} \right] (t+n) \tag{8}$$

5　Scope to Use Artificial Intelligence and Data Science

Tools based on artificial intelligence can be used to analyze the coronavirus outbreak. It can also be used to predict the nature of spread. These tools, in general, require reasonable amount of data with variety. Presently, the availability of coronavirus outbreak data is the key concern. Existing artificial intelligence-based models are not capable enough to analyze and predict about the coronavirus outbreak. As the coronavirus outbreak is nonlinear in nature and varying with time, so the developed artificial intelligence-based model should be based on the multitudinal and multi-modal data. To make the model or system more robust, one can explore the concepts of data science to generate the knowledge. Based on this knowledge representation, the model or system can be evolved.

6　Conclusion

As incubation period of coronavirus is of two weeks, it is difficult to predict anything initially. Rather, the preventive measures can be adopted for the avoidance of spread. Presented mathematical formulation is carried out on the basis of identified preventive and corrective measures and the constraints. Association and dependencies of these measures and constraints are also explored from the evaluation of positive cases, mortality, transmission rate, recovery and prediction of peak time of spread. This mathematical formulation can be applied with certain time intervals to evaluate, predict and optimize the mentioned objectives with some empirical estimation of the constraint parameters and their weight factor values. Presently, the evaluation has not been carried out, but the data from the reliable sources like John Hopkins University can be used for the evaluation. Very soon the evaluation of proposed mathematical formulation will be carried out. This leads for the scope of improvement in the presented mathematical formulation.

References

1. World Health Organization. Coronavirus. World Health Organization, cited April 15, 2020. Available: https://www.who.int/health-topics/coronavirus
2. International Committee on Taxonomy of Viruses, cited April 15, 2020. Available: https://talk.ictvonline.org/
3. Gorbalenya, A. E., Baker, S. C., Baric, R. S., et al. (2020). The species Severe acute respiratory syndrome-related coronavirus: classifying 2019-nCoV and naming it SARS-CoV-2. *Nat Microbiol, 5,* 536–544. https://doi.org/10.1038/s41564-020-0695-z.
4. Zhou, P., Yang, X. L., Wang, X. G., Hu, B., Zhang, L., Zhang, W., et al. (2020). A pneumonia outbreak associated with a new coronavirus of probable bat origin. *Nature, 579,* 270–273. https://doi.org/10.1038/s41586-020-2012-7.
5. Huang, C., Wang, Y., Li, X., Ren, L., Zhao, J., Hu, Y., et al. (2020). Clinical features of patients infected with 2019 novel coronavirus in Wuhan, China. *The Lancet, 395,* 497–506. https://doi.org/10.1016/S0140-6736(20)30183-5.
6. Chan, J. F., Yuan, S., Kok, K. H., To, K. K., Chu, H., Yang, J., et al. (2020). A familial cluster of pneumonia associated with the 2019 novel coronavirus indicating personto-person transmission: a study of a family cluster. *The Lancet, 395,* 514–523. https://doi.org/10.1016/S0140-6736(20)30154-9.
7. Zhu N, Zhang D, Wang W, Li X, Yang B, Song J, et al. (2020) A novel coronavirus from patients with pneumonia in China, 2019. N Engl J Med: 727-733. https://doi.org/10.1056/NEJMoa2001017
8. Bogoch II, Watts A, Thomas-Bachli A, Huber C, Kraemer MUG, Khan K (2020) Pneumonia of unknown etiology in Wuhan, China: Potential for International Spread Via Commercial Air Travel. J Travel Med: 1-3. https://doi.org/10.1093/jtm/taaa008
9. Q&A on coronaviruses (COVID-19), cited April 8, 2020. Available: https://www.who.int/news-room/q-a-detail/q-a-coronaviruses
10. Stehlé, J., Voirin, N., Barrat, A., Cattuto, C., Colizza, V., Isella, L., et al. (2011). Simulation of an SEIR infectious disease model on the dynamic contact network of conference attendees. *BMC Medicine, 9,* 87.
11. Fisman, D., Khoo, E., & Tuite, A. (2014). Early epidemic dynamics of the west african 2014 ebola outbreak: estimates derived with a simple two-parameter model. *PLoS Curr., 6,* 6.
12. Das D, Santosh KC, Pal U (2020) Truncated Inception Net: COVID-19 Outbreak Screening using Chest X-rays, DOI:https://doi.org/10.21203/rs.3.rs-20795/v1
13. Mukherjee H, Ghosh S, Dhar A, Obaidullah SM, Santosh KC, Roy K (2020) Shallow Convolutional Neural Network for COVID-19 Outbreak Screening using Chest X-rays https://doi.org/10.36227/techrxiv.12156522.v1

14. Rajinikanth V, Dey N, Raj ANJ, Hassanien AE, Santosh KC, Raja N (2020) Harmony-Search and Otsu based System for Coronavirus Disease (COVID-19) Detection using Lung CT Scan Images. arXiv preprint arXiv:2004.03431.
15. Santosh, K. C. (2020). AI-Driven Tools for Coronavirus Outbreak: Need of Active Learning and Cross-Population Train/Test Models on Multitudinal/Multimodal Data. *Journal of Medical Systems, 44,* 93. https://doi.org/10.1007/s10916-020-01562-1.
16. Fong SJ, Li G, Dey N, Crespo RG, Herrera-Viedma E (2020) Finding an accurate early forecasting model from small dataset: A case of 2019-ncov novel coronavirus outbreak. arXiv preprint arXiv:2003.10776.
17. Fong SJ, Li G, Dey N, Crespo RG, Herrera-Viedma E (2020) Composite Monte Carlo decision making under high uncertainty of novel coronavirus epidemic using hybridized deep learning and fuzzy rule induction. Applied Soft Computing, 106282.
18. Coronavirus disease (COVID-19) outbreak situation, cited April 14, 2020. Available: https://www.who.int/emergencies/diseases/novel-coronavirus-2019
19. COVID-19 India, cited April 14, 2020. Available: https://www.mohfw.gov.in/

AI-Enabled Framework to Prevent COVID-19 from Further Spreading

Dalip and Deepika

Abstract The first case of COVID-19 was detected in Wuhan the city of China and now it has been spread over more than 100 countries. Due to this epidemic situation, the World Health Organization declares emergency in various cities and countries which causes an outbreak for COVID-19 that leads to control this virus spread. AI plays a significant role to control the COVID-19 a pandemic disease. This chapter explains an automated Artificial Intelligence Enabled (AIE) framework which is designed to control the further spread of the novel coronavirus. Artificial intelligence (AI) is used to address about the current disease coronavirus if applied in an innovative way. The main motive of this chapter suggested that AI is merged with the latest technologies like machine learning (ML) and Global Positioning System (GPS) which are used to design an innovative automation system which is used to control the further spreading of coronavirus. For experimental results, the concept of AIE framework is designed by considering the scenario of urban and rural regions of the state of Haryana(India). The comparative analysis of AIE with traditional frameworks is shown in Table 1 which defines the novelty and efficiency of designed framework. Finally on the basis of this innovative AIE-designed automation system, the 98 and 97% accuracy is achieved in urban and rural regions respectively. Finally, we can conclude that this automated system is fully utilized and works efficiently to control and prevent the further spreading of this novel epidemic coronavirus.

Keywords Artificial intelligence · COVID-19 · Coronavirus · Automation system · GPS · Regions · Locations · Machine learning

Dalip (✉) · Deepika
M.M. Institute of Computer Technology and Business Management, Maharishi Markandeshwar (Deemed to be University), Mullana–Ambala, Haryana, India
e-mail: dalipkamboj65@gmail.com

Deepika
e-mail: deepikalibra@gmail.com

© The Author(s), under exclusive license to Springer Nature Singapore Pte Ltd. 2020   29
A. Joshi et al. (eds.), *Intelligent Systems and Methods to Combat Covid-19*,
SpringerBriefs in Computational Intelligence,
https://doi.org/10.1007/978-981-15-6572-4_4

1 Introduction

This novel coronavirus (COVID-19) threats a human life across all over the world. As per the existing data analytics, total number [6] of COVID-19 cases are 2,192,974, total deaths are 147,376, total recovered are 554,676, total active are 1,490,922 and total serious critical are 56,566 by the time of writing this chapter. It also brings huge economic losses along with the serious threats to human lives and proves to be an infectious disease. A group of experts is working toward the development of vaccines against COVID-19 but no vaccine is founded for coronavirus till date. This epidemic virus is spread from the Wuhan which acts as an origin of this pandemic disease and now spread almost in the entire globe over more than 100 countries. China takes the first initiative to implement preventive measures to control this virus as this country has strong medical background and has best medical facilities. There are different technologies like artificial intelligence (AI), Internet of Things (IoT) and data science that are used to track and fight against this disease [1]. The innovative applications can be designed with the help of AI to track and fight against COVID-19 such as location tracking and geo-fencing are used to track the infected peoples. By analyzing news reports, social media platforms and government documents AI can be used to identify, track and forecast outbreaks. AI designed models are used to help medical professional to a greater extent as huge chances are there to get them infected from this disease as they are intact contact with the infected persons. Another technology is drones which helps the medical workers to protect themselves from this infected disease in order to provide the medical supplies to their patients in a safest way without going in contact with the infected person. A robotics application of an AI can protect our homes, buildings, streets and cities from this virus and this disease cannot harm robots so they are used to accomplished many tasks such as cleaning, sterilizing, delivering food and provide medical facilities to the patients to avoid the human to human interaction. Robots are also utilized by the police officials in an effective way in order to protect them from this virus by avoiding the regular public interaction. So with these types of AI systems the police persons, medicated staff and sweepers can protect themselves. The IoT-based patient care system can help to measure their temperatures and upload the measurements with their mobile devices to the cloud for further analysis. Due to the lack of AI-enabled automated models, therefore an AIE automated framework is designed by using the existing technologies which helps us to control and prevent the further spread of this novel epidemic coronavirus. The proposed framework automatically calculates the fuzzy weight and threshold values for decision making.

The rest of the chapter is categorized as follows. Sect. 2 discussed about the related work and elaborates the contribution of different researchers over COVID-19. Motivation and contribution are explained in Sect. 3. A novel methodology of the proposed framework is shown in Sect. 4. The results and discussion are analysis in Sect. 5. At last, the conclusion is present in Sect. 6.

2 Background

The World Health Organization (WHO) [1] has been declared coronavirus an epidemic contagious disease that transmit from human to human very rapidly which becomes a danger for human life in all the age groups. So, if the rate of transmission between human to human is reduced like 0.25 then we can control this virus at some extent [7]. This virus spread rapidly across various countries and among the whole world and also proves to be a threat for the global health and for the economy as well. This virus named as novel coronavirus disease COVID-2019 [1] which states a total number of 80,868 confirmed cases and 3,101 deaths [6] in Chinese mainland by National Health Commission of China by March 8, 2020. In the early stage of this virus, no one thinks about this epidemic situation comes and this will rise to an emergency in China. To outbreak this pandemic, the Chinese officials take some preventive and strict actions to restrict their all resources especially traveling, business and schools. The lockdown and curfew need to be implemented to save the human lives and to outbreak this pandemic. It becomes a difficult task to know about the time span of this outbreak of coronavirus. For this, some automated models are need to be designed with the help of some existing models and latest technologies. With the help of existing studies, various models of explainable AI are there that explains how people define, generate, select, present and evaluate explanations [2]. The disease spread simulation model and contact tracking system are helpful to prevent and control this infectious disease [3]. These contact tracking system are helpful for the medical [5] professionals to identify the infected and high-risk peoples from this disease and to locate and then isolate them so that they cannot further spread this virus among other human beings [4]. The other innovative techniques like composite Monte-Carlo model (CMC) uses GROOMS methodology [7], deep learning and various soft computing algorithms and techniques like Fuzzy Rule Induction, BFGS and PNN that provides efficient results for decision support. As a result, the data collected by the agencies of China government using the CMC methodology on this epidemic disease COVID-19 are superior than their earlier methods. The forecasting model [8] uses data mining and machine learning concepts which uses Polynomial Neural Network with Corrective Feedback (PNN + CF) which calculate the prediction time with lower error rates and becomes a best technique to determine the critical times of this disease outbreak. The forecasting model is one of the best alternatives to deal with the future epidemics. It is important to predict the lifetime of this virus in early stages so that preventive measures should be taken to spread this virus like schools, commercial, etc. are closed. Artificial intelligence (AI) are also deployed with machine learning algorithms, test models and test cases which are used for data analysis and decision-making processes sets a new dimensions in healthcare. AI-driven tools are implemented during the time of data collection where active learning [9] is to be deployed with it. It means AI tools are used to determine this disease outbreak forecast time which spread all over the globe and is useful to prevent this coronavirus further spread.

To prevent and control this epidemic disease, an AI-based contact tracing systems are suggested. The motivation and contributions of the AIE framework are explained in the next section.

3 Motivation and Contributions

The existing studies present different research work on COVID-19 such as comparative analysis, innovative techniques, models and AI-based decision-making systems, etc. The challenge of designing an efficient framework is that there are lack of AI designed enabled automation systems for coronavirus which inspires us to design the Artificial Intelligence Enabled (AIE) automated framework that helps to control and prevents COVID-19 from further spreading. The proposed methodology is based on face and full body detection that prevent coronavirus spread by tracing the camera locations in both the urban and rural regions; also send the alerts and notifications at authorized center on rigid time.

4 A Novel Methodology

A novel framework is designed which helps to detect the COVID-19 infected persons from both the rural and urban regions on different times and locations by using preventive measures. The proposed system automatically divides the regions into three clusters or zones based on their fuzzy weights and also set the threshold values to the movement attributes. The movement attributes are those which are useful to decide the parameter for movement in lockdown situations. The zones categorization is done on the basis of more, less and not affected with COVID-19 as they are considered as RED, ORANGE and GREEN zones, respectively. The color label of these zones will depend on their fuzzy weights which will automatically update.

The fuzzy weights assigned in these zones on the basis of the occurrence of COVID-19 causes. The RED zone is known as hot spotted zones; there will be no movement of public and services in between and full lockdown applicable. In ORANGE zones, there is partial movement of public and services with some conditions. In GREEN zones, there is a full movement of public and services under government guidelines. The full body and face detection module is implemented for screening the peoples and automatically detect persons those who are not follow the lockdown rules. The screening of the public is done on their gestures. If the gestures of the detected peoples are normal (no gestures of cough, cold and fever) than screening test will be negative and no action will be taken against those but if the gestures of the detected peoples are abnormal (gestures of cough, cold and fever) than screening test result will be positive and designed system send their location automatically at the authorized centers and government can take necessary action for their quarantine. There are three preventive measures which are to be taken for

Table 1 Comparative analysis between traditional framework and novel AIE framework for uniqueness

Framework components	Traditional framework	Novel AIE framework
Automation	Partially	Fully
Qualitative division	No	Yes
Coverage area	Urban only	Both urban and rural
Fuzzy weight assignment	No	Yes
Dynamically infected zone division	No	Yes

COVID-19 are social distancing, avoid social gathering and to wear face mask. The designed system automatically detects the person who violates these safety measures. If the safety measures conditions are fulfilled than no action will be taken, otherwise it sends the location to the authorized centers. It also sends alert notifications on time to the village authorities regarding those persons who disobey the safety measures given by the government. The uniqueness of the proposed system is shown in Table 1. For comparative analysis, the different parameters are taken. The AIE framework is a fully automated system which provides the accurate qualitative information on time about the infected person such as "more infected", "infected", "less infected" and "not infected" depends on their fuzzy score. It also tracks and locates the specific information of the infected people on the map and also provides the history of recently contacted persons with infected one. Geo-fencing provision is also used here which informs the authorized center and users also if any infected person leaves the isolation ward and try to enter in the fencing zone. India is primarily an agricultural country. During lockdown situations, the government of any country cannot stop the agriculture work for a long time. Therefore, there are more chances of COVID-19 spread in rural regions.

The proposed framework is also very helpful in rural regions. The system can monitor the safety measures against COVID-19 using drone technology. The designed system sends the alerts to the authorized centers in case of framers and laborers violate the safety measures against COVID-19. So that necessary action would be taken by authority on time. The application software AIE is implemented in Python programming language using Haar Cascades classifiers.

5 Results and Discussion

The designed system is tested over both the regions (Urban and Rural) on different locations, different dates and times. On x-axis, the first, second and third rows indicate locations, starting time and ending time, respectively.

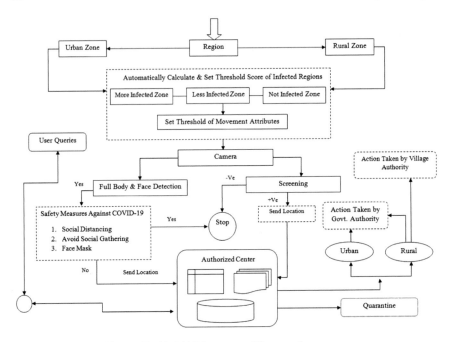

Fig. 1 Artificial Intelligence Enabled (AIE) automated framework

The given calculations are obtained up to writing this chapter during the lockdown period for the best results. Figure 2 shows the total number of cases detected for the different safety measures against COVID-19 on different locations and time periods automatically in urban regions. The 98% rate of accuracy is achieved by the AIE model in urban regions as shown in Fig. 2. Similarly, Fig. 3 showcases the total no. of infected cases for different safety measures automatically against COVID-19 on different locations and the time period in the rural region. The rate of accuracy measured by the AIE model is 97% in rural regions.

6 Conclusion

In this chapter, the automated AIE framework is designed on the basis of some existing models. After the analysis and study of some relevant and important findings from the existing research using the AI technology against COVID-19 which have been provided some insight into how this work can be used in an explainable designed framework, it has been quite cleared from Table 1 some unique components of the designed framework make it unique and more efficient. The AIE model can replicate its role in helping to control against the spread of COVID-19 pandemic in an efficient way with (97–98) % rate of accuracy.

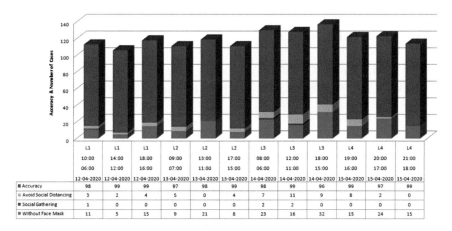

Fig. 2 Accuracy of AIE model in urban regions at different locations

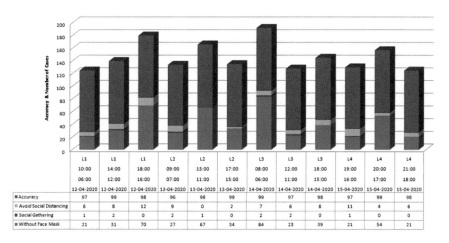

Fig. 3 Accuracy of AIE model in rural regions at different locations

References

1. Zhou, M., Zhang, X., & Qu, J. (2020). Coronavirus disease 2019 (COVID-19): A clinical update. *Frontiers in Medicine.* https://doi.org/10.1007/s11684-020-0767-8.
2. Miller, T. (2019). Explanation in artificial intelligence: Insights from the social sciences. *Artificial Intelligence, 267,* 1–38.
3. Tsui, K., Wong, Z. S., Goldsman, D., & Edesess, M. (2013). Tracking infectious disease spread for global pandemic containment. *IEEE Intelligent Systems, 28*(6), 60–64.
4. Chen, H., Yang, B., Pei, H., & Liu, J. (2018). Next generation technology for epidemic prevention and control: Data-driven contact tracking. *IEEE Access,* 1–1. https://doi.org/10.1109/access.2018.2882915.
5. Lupia, T., Scabini, S., Pinna, S. M., Di Perri, G., De Rosa, F. G., & Corcione, S. (2020). 2019 novel coronavirus (2019-nCoV) outbreak: A new challenge. *Journal of Global Antimicrobial Resistance, 21,* 22–27.

6. https://www.worldometers.info/coronavirus/#countries.
7. Fong, S. J., Li, G., Dey, N., Crespo, R. G., & Herrera-Viedma, E. (2020). Composite Monte Carlo decision making under high uncertainty of novel coronavirus epidemic using hybridized deep learning and fuzzy rule induction. *Applied Soft Computing*. https://doi.org/10.1016/j.asoc.2020.106282.
8. Fong, S. J., Li, G., Dey, N., Crespo, R. G., & Herrera-Viedma, E. (2020). Finding an accurate early forecasting model from small dataset: A case of 2019-nCoV novel coronavirus outbreak. *International Journal of Interactive Multimedia and Artificial Intelligence, Special Issue on Soft Computing, 6*(1), 132–140. https://doi.org/10.9781/ijimai.2020.02.002.
9. Santosh, K. C. (2020). AI-driven tools for coronavirus outbreak: Need of active learning and cross-population train/test models on multitudinal/multimodal data. *Journal of Medical Systems*. https://doi.org/10.1007/s10916-020-01562-1.

Artificial Intelligence-Enabled Robotic Drones for COVID-19 Outbreak

Dharm Singh Jat and Charu Singh

Abstract Artificial intelligence (AI) can help to address coronavirus if applied creatively. Artificial intelligence training models to deal with COVID-19 are having challenges as historical data is still not available. Drones and robots equipped with IoT devices provide raw data that needs computing analysis to make that data meaningful and actionable without human involvement. The power of AI and edge computing lies in its ability to process a massive amount of data at breakneck speed and improving efficiency. It enables big data analytics and deployment of algorithm and transmission of data across edge and cloud. This chapter presents how current artificial intelligence enables robotic drone applications and network connectivity is used to improve their performance and increase efficiency in various situations to fight COVID-19. Further, it provides an in-depth review and analysis of literature on related work on COVID-19 outbreak. It also gives the necessary background for future research in edge intelligence, AI-enabled robotic drone and intelligent networks.

Keywords Artificial intelligence · COVID-19 · 5G · Edge computing · Robotic drone

1 Introduction

Artificial Intelligence (AI) is the fourth industrial revolution technology in the current and developing environment. People from the various fields are trying to implement AI to solve their problems. Artificial intelligence has not yet been impactful to fight COVID-19 outbreak due to massive and noisy data. It is up to us to identify new and innovative ways to leverage what AI can do. Artificial intelligence-enabled drones

D. S. Jat (✉)
Namibia University of Science and Technology, Windhoek, Namibia
e-mail: dsingh@nust.na

C. Singh
University of Southern California, Los Angeles, CA, USA
e-mail: charusin@usc.edu

© The Author(s), under exclusive license to Springer Nature Singapore Pte Ltd. 2020   37
A. Joshi et al. (eds.), *Intelligent Systems and Methods to Combat Covid-19*,
SpringerBriefs in Computational Intelligence,
https://doi.org/10.1007/978-981-15-6572-4_5

can be useful to fight COVID-19 by the monitoring system and can process the captured data and report back in real time.

Self-directed drones pose many challenges like lack of wireless bandwidth, limited processing capacity, non-availability of sufficient power, accuracy and latency for real-time applications [1]. In this study, the experimental results describe that the integration of edge computing devices and drones processing power can save the essential wireless bandwidth requirement and therefore increase throughput, improve scalability and decrease latency for sensitive application applications [1]. Artificial intelligence software can be useful to guide drone for collecting the raw data and process it into actionable insights for emergency teams including doctor, police, etc., during COVID-19 or similar situation [2].

The study presents a framework that determines the optimal location of the distribution centre in a disaster-affected region for low-cost drones for emergency supply and services. The drones may not be useful for densely and sparsely population centres due to drone routing limitations. Further study also do not consider power constraints and assume fully charged battery will be available for drones during distribution [3]. A study related to edge intelligence provides insights for possible future research in AI at the edge [4]. The rapid advancement of communication technologies and Internet of things devices (IoTs) generates a billion of data bytes at the network edge. Therefore, there is a high demand for integrated AI and edge computing to process and analyse the data at the edge. Further, the study describes artificial intelligence on edge as well as intelligence-enabled edge computing. The edge intelligence is in the early stage and has attracted more and more researchers, organisations and industries to get involved in research in this area [4].

2 Motivation and Contributions

Experts recognised a novel coronavirus (nCoV) in December 2019 in China and governments and authorities all over the world are facing challenges to control COVID-19 outbreak [5]. A study states that there is a need to predict the epidemic outbreak for timely decision and measures, including closing universities, schools, international and interstate borders and suspending crowded community services and customers [6]. For post-COVID-19 outbreak, the suitable training models for AI-driven tools were discussed and also mentioned that many machine learning (ML) algorithms are useful for decision-making related to medical procedures and treatments and to identify infested COVID-19 cases [7].

More researches recently published on chest X-rays for detection of infested COVID-19 cases. One of the research suggested the method based on convolutional neural network for automatic chest X-rays for detection of infested COVID-19 [8]. A study proposed an image-assisted system to extract information from lung CT scans of COVID-19 infected cases. It will also assist the pulmonologist in helping in developing the best treatment plan [9]. X-ray imaging techniques are cheaper than CT scan systems. Therefore, a study suggested Truncated Inception Net deep learning model is used to detect infested COVID-19 positive cases using chest X-rays [10].

Most of the researches have been conducted for COVID-19 outbreak which focuses on chest X-rays detection of infested COVID-19 cases [5–10].

According to the researchers' best knowledge, a few published literature exists on artificial intelligence-enabled robotic drones technology; therefore, there is a gap in research for drones technology and communication for COVID-19 outbreak.

This study describes how artificial intelligence-enabled robotic drones are being used to improve their performance and increase efficiency in various situations during and post-COVID-19 outbreak. In COVID-19 outbreak, the intelligent drone can be used to recognise people of interest from the large gathering. Moreover, the problem of power and computing can be solved by implementing the edge computing devices so that drones can offload their data for pre-processing and receive desired action to be taken.

In summary, this chapter provides an in-depth review of the literature on artificial intelligence-enabled robotic drone used to fight COVID-19 and other similar scenarios. The chapter also describes AI-enabled intelligent networks, future generation networks (5G) and intelligent edge.

3   Related Work on COVID-19 Outbreak

These days, drone technology is being used in various applications, including natural disaster relief, defence, security, construction, agriculture, etc. Individuals and small organisations cannot afford as such systems are bulky and expensive. The AI-enabled drone can be used for the monitoring system as they can now process what they record and report back in real time. AI can be useful to guide the drone to capture raw data and provide it for police, doctors and other emergency teams for the action to be taken. The AI-powered drone can be used to identify the hotspot areas during COVID-19 outbreak.

More research work is needed in the area related technology to make drones a valuable and reliable source of information for various organisations. Drones and other sensor-equipped devices provide raw data which requires computing analysis to make that data meaningful and actionable without human involvement. Edge computing devices and IoT applications enable analytics, machine learning, and seamless deployment of algorithm and transmission of data across the edge and the cloud [11].

3.1 Robotic Technology

Intelligent robots are progressively being used in various fields. The study suggested optimal methods for the control of mobile robots with the help of artificial intelligence technology. Further, the study implemented this AI technology for traffic control robot modelling and robotic sprinkler system in the field of irrigation. This developed mechanism can also be used for the algorithm design of mobile robots in other applications [12]. A police robot has been used to monitor areas of Tunisia's capital, Tunis, to make sure that people are following a coronavirus lockdown. This robot can help to reduce physical contact between police and residents/patients suffering from COVID-19 [13].

China is progressively using robotic technology and artificial intelligence (AI) during these exceptional times. This technology is used in the form of disinfecting robots, thermal camera-equipped drones, etc., to fight coronavirus. During the peak outbreak of the disease in China, smart helmets, disinfecting robots, and advanced facial recognition software are being used to fight against COVID-19 [14]. Many Chinese companies have innovated automated technologies for contact-free delivery, spraying sanitizers and executing necessary diagnostic tasks to reduce the spread of the infection. In Shenzhen city, MicroMultiCopter drones are also being deployed to transport medical samples and also to perform thermal imaging [14].

3.2 Drones Against COVID-19

Nowadays, mini-unmanned aerial vehicles (UAVs) called drones are being used in many application related to agriculture, defence, communications, surveillance, public services, photography due to several advantages like low cost, low power requirement, easy to transport, etc. These drones can also provide real-time activities by transmitting real-time video streaming and can be used to pose severe outbreak to community security like situational awareness information for COVID-19 outbreak.

The main problems faced by implementing drones in public residence are a direct physical attack on building, property, people and other infrastructure. Additionally, the research suggested a deep learning-based method to identify the possible illegal drones in real time in the area of interest [15]. The study proposed a model for drone crowdsourcing and demonstrated the use of drone in a fire situation at the island. In such a situation, with the help of drone and devices, people can be located who are stuck. Drones are having limited resources and can carry limited weight and lightweight battery only. Some applications also require multiple drones, which are working in a coordinated manner. Therefore, the combination of additional resources (edge devices) beyond the drone capability and multiple drown can overcome these limitations [16].

The study presents the application of drones in precision agriculture farming. The farmer can control the overall area of the attacked plants or observe the activities of parasites moving among plants by drones equipped with the camera [17]. In agriculture, plant disease can be identified in early stage by using drones together with camera and the global positioning system (GPS) device. This early detection will help in stopping the infection from the crop. By implementing the Internet of things (IoT) devices and drone together, real-time data can be gathered and analysed with the help of image processing algorithm which performs the crop classification and disease detection [18].

A similar drone was deployed to sanitise the hotspots of COVID-19 by spraying a 1% sodium hypochlorite solution as a disinfectant over the locality by the South Delhi Municipal Corporation (SMDC) in India [19]. To control the spread of the virus, Delhi is under lockdown, and no public transport, including private buses, taxis and autorickshaws are allowed to ply on the roads. Delhi police make use of drones to monitor the situation in various areas, during the complete lockdown in Delhi [20]. Networked mobile robotics integrated with cameras are using in unmanned aerial vehicles (UAVs) and remotely steered aircraft systems to combat COVID-19 in improving responses to humanitarian emergencies, health monitoring and to detect the infectious and respiratory conditions which include monitoring body temperatures, heartbeats and respiratory rates [21].

Apart from robots and drones, China has also deployed many sophisticated surveillance mechanisms to keep a check on infested individuals and impose quarantines. Across China facial recognition cameras are ubiquitous. Some Chinese companies have introduced AI-enabled temperature detection systems and also to trace the people without masks [14].

3.3 AI-Enabled Intelligent Networks

Today 5G provides an economical solution for collecting and analysing data for real-time applications. AI techniques can improve automation to manage robotic drones, IoT connected devices and solve the problems that arise from 5G use cases and network complexity. Today's current mobile networks are providing services to the robotic drones in the low-altitude airspace only. 5G networks are capable of providing efficient mobile wireless connectivity for large-scale drone placements for various applications [22]. The integration of IoT and 5G technologies, operation and maintenance of communication networks, and the various industrial applications are facing many challenges. Artificial intelligence (AI) technology-based models have capabilities such as high computing massive data analysis, for network operation, management and maintenance in the future generation of wireless networks (5G) era [23].

For a real-time sensitive application like robotic drones application for COVID-19 outbreak, there is a need for reliable, low latency communications and ubiquitous connectivity with robotic drones. 5G next-generation wireless networks promise enhanced mobile broadband (eMBB), ultra-reliable low latency communications

(URLLC) and massive machine-type communications (mMTC) in a real-time application and dynamic environment. Data-driven functions and communication in 5G wireless networks can be empowered by using the concepts of machine learning across the wireless edge and core infrastructure [24].

Machine learning which is the subset of artificial intelligence (AI) has done a remarkable job in the communication technologies and can help telecom industries to optimise their investment and helpful in planning and smart slicing of 5G network. In the deployment of 5G wireless networks, AI-enabled edge is essential to minimise the cost. Strategy analytics predicts that the integration of artificial intelligence (AI) and edge computing technologies will be beneficial to deliver 5G connectivity as promised to improve the return on investment (ROI) [25].

3.4 5G: Coronavirus Outbreak

In the future, there will be a massive demand for high definition video and high resolution for mobile communication. The requirement for mobile broadband connectivity will continue to increase as the things around us become more connected.

The availability of lower bandwidth in 2G communication systems did not fulfil the need for immediate requirement of mobile Internet users. This led to a demand for new upgraded 3G standards, which advanced to provide fast data rate services and more bandwidth available for voice communication. Further, the 4G mobile communication system was developed to provide a high data rate service for multimedia communication. Groupe Speciale Mobile (GSM) later called as Global System for Mobile Telecommunication has provided mobile communications since 1991 to the world. In 2019, according to the GSM Association (GSMA) Intelligence, 4G long-term evolution (LTE) is also essential mobile network technology to support higher peak bit rates worldwide, and more than three billion number of connections worldwide.

Therefore, 1G provides only voice communication, 2G improves voice quality and provides a text messaging, 3G offers integrated voice, and affordable mobile Internet and 4G provides high data rate transmission for mobile multimedia communication. With the anticipated growth of the Internet of things (IoTs) and smart devices in future, there will be more users, more diverse range of device types than ever before.

Moreover, an emergency like COVID-19 outbreak will require low latency, high bandwidth, improved reliability and long battery life for devices like drones, robots, etc. All 4G LTE evolution will not be enough to handle this new wave of heterogeneous big data traffic. Therefore, there is a need for the upgraded new generation (5G) radio system and network architecture for the availability of high data rate broadband network and ultra-robust and low latency connectivity to connect people of everything. IoT applications in various fields are likely to be the main driver for further growth of WiFi and cellular communication. Therefore, IoTs applications will enable the devices like drones, robot, health devices etc., to interact and share data in real time. Nowadays, the network connects human, but in future 5G systems will be about people of things and become more and more connected every day.

Deploying wired broadband networks requires high investment, and it is not viable for least densely populated countries like Namibia. The estimated population density of Namibia is 2.6 persons per km^2 [26]. Fixed wireless access (FWA) networks can be used for more cost-effective and high-speed broadband networks installation.

WiMAX or LTE fixed wireless access networks are using for last-mile connectivity for many years, but the speed is slow in comparison with the wired high-speed broadband network. 5G communication also called as millimetre-wave communication is being considered for the use of above 6 GHz and the frequency bands are mentioned as the millimetre band (mm-band). Now by using 5G, the speed of FWA networks is comparable to the fibre network [27]. For rural area FWA networks, using below 6 GHz spectrums band can be used for broader coverage by applying massive MIMO technologies.

These days' people also believe that 5G radiation is the cause of coronavirus outbreak. Keri Hilson thinks that the cause of the coronavirus outbreak is due to 5G radiation [28]. The assumption behind this is that the Wuhan is the first city in China with 5G connectivity. However, at the time of COVID-19 spread, Wuhan was not the only city to have 5G connectivity, several other cities were also having 5G connectivity. People also assume that 5G harms the immune system of human beings. 5G is not accelerating the spread of the new coronavirus as there is no scientific evidence to support the negative impact on the immune system [29]. The statement related to the spread of the new coronavirus is incorrect as 5G wireless connectivity is based on radio frequency and therefore does not produce any type of viruses.

3.5   5G: COVID-19 Affected Africa

People also believe that COVID-19 has not affected Africa as it is "Not a 5G region" [28]. This statement is not valid, and 5G wireless networks are not the cause that Africa has not been affected by COVID-19. According to the report released by the World Health Organisation (WHO), Regional Office for Africa reported that COVID-19 is spreading nearly in every country. Around 17,000 COVID-19 positive cases and 900 deaths across the Africa continent as on 16 April 2020 were reported. South Africa is the country which has a severe outbreak of new coronavirus, while cases are still increasing in West and Central Africa [30].

African countries took preventive measures at the very initial stage of COVID-19 spread [31]. Appropriate precautionary measures were taken to deal with COVID-19 outbreak on time as soon as WHO declared COVID-19 as a global pandemic. The Republic of Namibia also took the appropriate precautionary measure to deal with COVID-19 as soon as two confirmed cases of COVID-19 were found on Namibian soil. President of Namibia immediately declared a State Emergency and took the measures which aim at curbing the spread of the disease and mainly to prevent the occurrence of local transmission [32].

4 Conclusion

This chapter provides an in-depth review and analysis of literature on related work on COVID-19 outbreak, robotic technology, drones used to fight COVID-19, AI-enabled intelligent networks, 5G: coronavirus outbreak and 5G: COVID-19 affected Africa. Artificial intelligence has not yet been found impactful to fight COVID-19 due to big and noisy data. Also, there is a lack of historical data on which to train AI models to fight COVID-19. Artificial intelligence and edge computing devices, including robots and drones, can contribute to the fight against COVID-19: early warning systems for disasters and social control. Massive and noisy data can also be filtered at the edge by implementing edge computing devices. The statement related to the spread of the new coronavirus is due to 5G technology is incorrect because it is based on radio frequency and does not create viruses. Also, there is no scientific evidence to support that 5G harms the immune system. To conclude, this chapter describes AI-enabled intelligent networks, future generation networks (5G) and intelligent edge.

References

1. Wang, J., et al. (2018). Bandwidth-efficient live video analytics for drones via edge computing. In *Proceedings of 2018 3rd ACM/IEEE Symposium on Edge Computing SEC 2018* (pp. 159–173).
2. International Telecommunication Union. (2019). *Artificial intelligence for good*. [Online]. Available: https://www.itu.int/en/mediacentre/backgrounders/Pages/artificial-intelligence-for-good.aspx.
3. Chowdhury, S., Emelogu, A., Marufuzzaman, M., Nurre, S. G., & Bian, L. (2017). Drones for disaster response and relief operations: A continuous approximation model. *International Journal of Production Economics, 188,* 167–184.
4. Deng, S., Zhao, H., Fang, W., Yin, J., Dustdar, S., & Zomaya, A. Y. (2020). Edge intelligence: The confluence of edge computing and artificial intelligence. *IEEE Internet of Things Journal, PP*(c), 1.
5. Fong, S. J., Li, G., Dey, N., Crespo, R. G., & Herrera-Viedma, E. (2020). Composite Monte Carlo decision making under high uncertainty of novel coronavirus epidemic using hybridized deep learning and fuzzy rule induction. *Applied Soft Computing,* 106282.
6. Fong, S. J., Li, G., Dey, N., Gonzalez-Crespo, R., & Herrera-Viedma, E. (2020). Finding an accurate early forecasting model from small dataset: A case of 2019-nCoV novel coronavirus outbreak. *International Journal of Interactive Multimedia and Artificial Intelligence, 6*(1), 132.
7. Santosh, K. C. (2020). AI-driven tools for coronavirus outbreak: Need of active learning and cross-population train/test models on multitudinal/multimodal data. *Journal of Medical Systems, 44*(5), 1–5.
8. Mukherjee, H., Ghosh, S., Dhar, A., & Obaidullah, S. (2019). Shallow convolutional neural network for COVID-19 outbreak screening using chest, 1–10.
9. Rajinikanth, V., Dey, N., Raj, A. N. J., Hassanien, A. E., Santosh, K. C., & Raja, N. S. M. (2020). Harmony-search and Otsu based system for coronavirus disease (COVID-19) detection using lung CT scan images.

10. Das, U. P. D., & Santosh, K. C. (2020). Truncated inception net: COVID-19 outbreak screening using chest X-rays. [Online]. Available: https://doi.org/10.21203/rs.3.rs-20795/v1.
11. Guttman, C. (2019). *Drone innovation turns to edge computing*. 2019 Nutanix, Inc. [Online]. Available: https://www.nutanix.com/theforecastbynutanix/technology/drone-innovation-turns-to-edge-computing%0A.
12. Irshat, K., Petr, R., & Irina, R. (2018). The selecting of artificial intelligence technology for control of mobile robots. In *International Multi-Conference on Industrial Engineering and Modern Technologies. FarEastCon 2018* (pp. 1–4).
13. Jawad, R. (2020). Coronavirus: Tunisia deploys police robot on lockdown patrol. [Online]. Available: https://www.bbc.com/news/world-africa-52148639.
14. Jakhar, P. (2020). Coronavirus: China's tech fights back. [Online]. Available: https://www.bbc.com/news/technology-51717164.
15. Chen, H., Wang, Z., & Zhang, L. (2020). Collaborative spectrum sensing for illegal drone detection: A deep learning-based image classification perspective. *China Communications, 17*(2), 81–92.
16. Alwateer, M., Loke, S. W., & Fernando, N. (2019). Enabling drone services: Drone crowdsourcing and drone scripting. *IEEE Access, 7,* 110035–110049.
17. Potrino, G., Palmieri, N., Antonello, V., & Serianni, A. (2018). Drones support in precision agriculture for fighting against parasites. In *2018 26th Telecommunications Forum, TELFOR 2018—Proceedings* (pp. 1–4).
18. Kitpo, N., & Inoue, M. (2018). Early rice disease detection and position mapping system using drone and IoT architecture. In *Proceedings—12th SEATUC Symposium SEATUC 2018* (p. 4).
19. IANS. (2020, April 2). Drone deployed to sanitize Nizamuddin Markaz, the 'epicentre' of COVID-19 outbreak. *The New Indian Express.*
20. Delhi police uses drone to monitor the situation amid lockdown. (2020, April 1). *ABP Live.* [Online]. Available: https://news.abplive.com/topic/drone.
21. Cozzens, T. (2020, March 26). Pandemic drones to monitor, detect those with COVID-19. [Online]. Available: https://www.gpsworld.com/draganfly-camera-and-uav-expertise-to-help-diagnose-coronavirus/#comments.
22. Takacs, A., Lin, X., Hayes, S., & Tejedor, E. (2018). Drones and networks: Ensuring safe and secure operations. *Ericsson White Paper,* 14.
23. *ZTE uSmartNet network intelligent solution.* ZTE Corporation. [Online]. Available: https://www.zte.com.cn/global/solutions/201905201711/201905201746/201906170947.
24. Chen, M., Challita, U., Saad, W., Yin, C., & Debbah, M. (2019). Artificial neural networks-based machine learning for wireless networks: A tutorial. *IEEE Communications Surveys & Tutorials, 21*(4), 3039–3071.
25. de Grimaldo, S. W. (2018). *AI + edge computing essential in the 5G era* (pp. 1–9).
26. *Census projected population.* The Government of Namibia. [Online]. Available: https://gov.na/population.
27. Samsung. (2018). *5G fixed wireless access.* Samsung Electronica Co., Ltd. [Online]. Available: https://images.samsung.com/is/content/samsung/p5/global/business/networks/insights/white-paper/samsung-5g-fwa/white-paper_samsung-5g-fixed-wireless-access.pdf.
28. Cedric "BIG CED" Thornton. *Keri Hilson believes the coronavirus outbreak may have been caused by 5G radiation.* [Online]. Available: https://www.blackenterprise.com/keri-hilson-believes-the-coronavirus-outbreak-may-have-been-caused-by-5g-radiation/.
29. Milan, A. (2020). Coronavirus UK: Why do people think 5G is responsible for the COVID-19 pandemic? *Metro, UK.* [Online]. Available: https://metro.co.uk/2020/04/02/coronavirus-uk-people-think-5g-responsible-covid-19-pandemic-12500019/?ito=cbshare.
30. World Health Organisation. *WHO, WFP and AU deliver critical supplies as COVID-19 accelerates in West and Central Africa.* [Online]. Available: http://whotogo-whoafroccmaster.newsweaver.com/JournalEnglishNewsletter/10dge3vjomny48iiujdam4?email=true&lang=en&a=11&p=56844493.

31. *African countries move from COVID-19 readiness to response as many confirm cases.* World Health Organization. [Online]. Available: https://www.afro.who.int/health-topics/coronavirus-covid-19.
32. President of the Republic of Namibia. (2020, March 28). *State of emergency—COVID-19 regulations: Namibian constitution, government gazette of the Republic of Namibia* (No. 7159). Windhoek, Republic of Namibia.

Understanding and Analysis of Enhanced COVID-19 Chest X-Ray Images

M. C. Hanumantharaju, V. N. Manjunath Aradhya,
and G. Hemantha Kumar

Abstract The 2019 coronavirus disease (COVID-19) with its origin in China has spread rapidly to other nations and infected millions of people. In this context, this paper proposes the development of algorithm that enhances the details of images and assists the doctors in knowing the exact location of affected area. The proposed technique improvises the most popular image enhancement algorithm, namely, multiscale retinex and adjusts the parameters to intensify the details of chest X-ray/CT images of COVID-19 patients. Multiscale retinex (MSR) is human perception-related enhancement algorithm which improves intensity, contrast, and sharpness in medical image through dynamic range compression. The proposed scheme improves the details of images and validates the resulting images using novel metric called wavelet energy. The proposed study is evaluated on images of COVID-19 patients have been obtained from the open-source GitHub repository. Considering the experimental result presented and performance metric, the proposed algorithm has provided important details to doctors in making right decision.

Keywords COVID-19 · Image enhancement · Improved multiscale retinex · Wavelet energy · X-ray/CT images

M. C. Hanumantharaju
Department of Electronics and Communication Engineering, BMS Institute of Technology and Management, Bengaluru, India
e-mail: mchanumantharaju@bmsit.in

V. N. Manjunath Aradhya (✉)
Department of Computer Applications, JSS Science and Technology University, Mysuru 570006, India
e-mail: aradhya@jssstuniv.in

G. Hemantha Kumar
Department of Studies in Computer Science, University of Mysore, Mysuru 570006, India
e-mail: ghk.2007@yahoo.com

© The Author(s), under exclusive license to Springer Nature Singapore Pte Ltd. 2020   47
A. Joshi et al. (eds.), *Intelligent Systems and Methods to Combat Covid-19*,
SpringerBriefs in Computational Intelligence,
https://doi.org/10.1007/978-981-15-6572-4_6

1 Introduction

Globally, nearly 3 million confirmed cases of COVID 2019 have been reported to World Health Organization (WHO) and more than 2,10,000 deaths as of April 28, 2020. We are seeing alarming acceleration in several countries and spread of virus to rural areas and can see clusters of cases and community spread in more than 16 countries. Pneumonia, headache, fever, dry cough, and breathing difficulties are the typical symptoms of the patients infected from this disease. Respiratory problem owing to alveolar damage (can be seen in chest CT images) and even death may be the result of this disease. With this outbreak, the question is with different testing methods and its efficiency at this level. With respect to the various tests available, radiological imaging can also help in diagnosing the COVID efficiently. Recently, it is noted that among radiological imaging data, assessment of disease through chest imaging is of great use in understanding and analysis of COVID-19 [1, 2]. Initial chest imaging reported abnormal findings in most of the patients of COVID 2019 [3]. It is also suggested that, imaging technique such as CT or X-ray is quite recommended for follow up in individuals who are recovering from COVID 2019 and can be effectively detected. Automated artificial intelligence models/tools are a must in order to categorize COVID-19 positive cases to non-positive and these tools can help in providing accurate results [2, 4]. Medical imaging system with deep architectures including shape and spatial relation features have been reported in the literature [5]. Interesting research works have been reported in recent past on COVID 2019 [6]. Image enhancement certainly assists physicians in detecting and diagnosis anomaly/abnormality in automated medical imaging systems and few recent works on image enhancements can be seen in [4, 7–13]. Variants of MSR algorithms can be seen in the literature recent past. Our previous works on retinex-based algorithm are reported in the literature. Using a popular particle swarm optimization (PSO) for color image enhancement based on MSR [14], medical image enhancement based on multi-rate sampling is addressed in [15]. Image quality metric plays an important role in design and evaluation process of imaging systems. In this connection, accurate objective criterion for assessing the performance of image enhancement algorithms is a concern.

The main contributions of this paper are: (i) we propose an improvised version of retinex algorithm for better analysis of COVID-19 chest X-ray/CT images. (ii) The resultant of the proposed algorithm may be used in diagnosis and assist the doctors and radiologists in detecting the spread of virus in chest and lower intestine part of human body effectively. (iii) Concept of wavelet energy is introduced for evaluation purpose. The remaining part of the paper is as follows: proposed methodology followed by experiment and critical analysis is shown in Sects. 2 and 3, respectively. Paper concludes in Sect. 4.

2 Proposed Methodology

The process of conversion from RGB to HSV space is much essential and resolves the gray world violation problem that exists in the traditional retinex algorithm. The HSV domain processing also avoids color shifting issues because the value or intensity channel is separated from chrominance component. The proposed improved multiscale retinex (MSR) algorithm is applied on the value component by preserving hue and saturation. Retinex is human perception based enhancement algorithm that improves intensity, contrast, and sharpness in medical image through dynamic range compression. The parameter of retinex algorithm varies adaptively depending on the intensity component and image depth. The improved image is validated using a wavelet energy metric [16] that reveal approximate and detail components. Approximate coefficients provide global enhanced information and detail coefficients convey sharpness of the image. The proposed framework exploits envelop-based retinex method [17] to obtain the illumination. In traditional retinex algorithm [18], illumination estimation is achieved by applying several Gaussians surround functions and produces the resultant image by processing the reflectance in the logarithmic domain.

2.1 Illumination Estimation

The proposed method assumes spatial smoothness in the original image and need of envelop is based on the technique proposed by Kimmel [19]. The computational complexity in the traditional retinex algorithm is mainly due to the log domain processing. This complication has been overcome here by processing each pixel directly instead of using logarithm. With the need of piecewise spatial smoothness in the original image, we concatenate the weighting function with the envelope and restrict the performance of the illumination around the boundaries and corners of an image. Because of spatial smoothness assumption in the original image, the derivative of illumination has to be minimized. In addition, we restrict that the illumination is close in order to achieve low reflectance. Based on these procedures, we model the cost operator and minimize its penalty using Eq. (1)

$$F(L(x, y)) = \int \left(\|\nabla L(x, y)\|^2 + \alpha \|L(x, y) - I(x, y)\|^2 \right) \mathrm{d}x \mathrm{d}y \qquad (1)$$

where ∇ specify first-order differential operator and $\|.\|$ operation retains positive values. Subsequently, we use cost-minimizing operation in descent gradient framework. Further, the iteration framework is formulated as given by Eq. (2)

$$L_j(x, y) = L_{j-1}(x, y) - \beta \cdot G \qquad (2)$$

where $L_j(x, y)$ and $L_{j-1}(x, y)$ denotes intensity images at jth step and $(j-1)$th step; β signify the step size, G denote gradient operator of $F(L(x, y))$

The gradient operator defined in [19] is given by

$$G = -\Delta L + \alpha(L - 1) \tag{3}$$

$$G \approx -L(x, y) * K_{\text{lap}}(x, y) + \alpha \cdot (L(x, y) - I(x, y)) \tag{4}$$

Here Δ the second-order Laplacian differential operator that is predicted as a convolution operation with the spatial filter.

Lastly, we formulate the equation to obtain the illumination.

$$L_j(x, y) = \max\{w(\nabla I) \cdot I(x, y) + (1 - w(\nabla I)) \cdot L_j(x, y) \cdot I(x, y)\} \tag{5}$$

$$w(\nabla I) = \begin{cases} w_0, & \text{if} \quad \nabla I > \text{Th} \\ w_0 \cdot \left(\frac{\nabla I}{\text{Th}}\right)^2, & \text{Otherwise} \end{cases} \tag{6}$$

$$\nabla I \approx \|I(x, y) * H(x, y)\| + \|I(x, y) * H^{\text{T}}(x, y)\| \tag{7}$$

where Th is the threshold, $H(x, y)$ indicates pyramid operator, $H^{\text{T}}(x, y)$ indicates the transpose of $H(x, y)$ used to make use of robust edge.

2.2 Estimation of Reflectance

In this work, estimation of reflection is realized by dividing the value and resulting lighting. The brightness adaptive change and depth image improvement are achieved by the following equations:

$$\Gamma(y) = N\left(\frac{L}{N}\right)^{k\left(1+\frac{y}{N}\right)} \tag{8}$$

$$\beta(r) = \exp\left(g\left(\frac{1}{1 + e^{-b \cdot \log r}} - \frac{1}{2}\right)\right) \tag{9}$$

where k ranges from 0 to 1, b ranges from 0 to 10 and g varies between 1 and 10; N value is 255.

2.3 Validation of Enhanced Using Wavelet Energy (WE) Metric

To evaluate the amount of improvement of the proposed framework, we employed WE as a metric. As the detailed coefficients increases, the depth of the image is better. The enhanced component of the image is verified using WE metric. The Daubechies wavelet transform is employed in the WE computation. The depth of the image appears to be better if the detailed coefficients are large than the input image. Approximate WE coefficients are used to improve overall information of the image. Higher the approximate coefficients than the input image, globally the enhanced image appears to be better. More information about WE can be seen in [16, 20].

3 Experiment Results and Comparative Analysis

In this part, we show the experiments and comparative analysis with standard well-known algorithm. We have conducted a number of experiments on more than 100 images from variety of COVID-19 database publically available in [21]. As it was found from the experimental results that proposed scheme reconstructs the images with improved quality, more visual details and improved appearance. The proposed enhancement scheme is mainly used by doctors, radiologists, and researchers in order to make right decisions. Figure 1 shows the experimental results obtained for various X-ray/CT scan images. Figure 1a shows the original X-ray/CT images of COVID 2019 patients of resolution 1024 × 768. Figure 1b shows the results obtained using NASA's multiscale retinex algorithm [18]. Figure 1c are the results of the proposed improved multiscale retinex algorithm. Corresponding histograms are also seen. The efficacy of the proposed algorithm is also tested and provided satisfactory results for CT scan images. In our experiments, we also opted CT scan images since these types of images assists in exact location of coronavirus spread. From the results, it is quite evident that the histogram plot of the enhanced image are tends toward the brightness area. Although histogram-based enhanced image analysis is subjective technique, objective techniques such as peak signal to noise ratio (PSNR), contrast enhancement performance (CEP), luminance enhancement performance (LEP), and wavelet energy (WE) are employed in this work. Table 1 shows the performance comparison for the set of images considered, which is based on PSNR, CEP, and LEP. From Table 1 it can be seen that the proposed algorithm is able to produce better results compared to existing MSRCR method. Table 2 shows the performance comparison applied on all four set of images (shown in Fig. 1) considered based on approximate and detailed wavelet energy. WE metric shows that the proposed method not only improves overall contrast of an image but also increases inner details in an image.

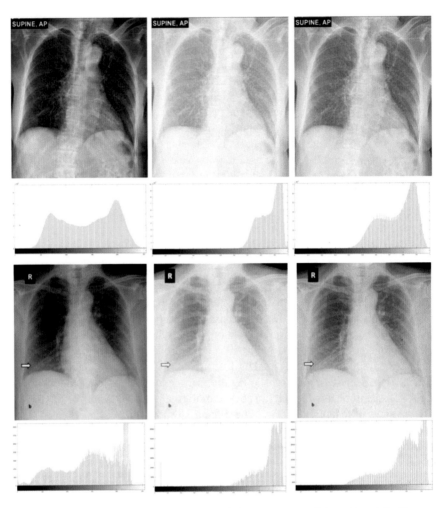

Fig. 1 Results for various images and its corresponding histogram. **a** Column 1—original images. **b** Column 2—multiscale retinex algorithm [18]. **c** Column 3—proposed algorithm

4 Discussion and Conclusion

Chest X-ray images are widely used to detect the COVID-19 positive cases mainly due to quick, easy, and accessible in all places. Radiologists recommend chest X-ray for the cases especially for the patients with non-transportable or difficult to move. The proposed adaptive retinex framework offers detailed enhanced results for both chest X-ray and CT scan images. Our scheme employs HSV domain-based retinex to separate chromatic component from intensity. The adaptive improved retinex method applied on value component of MSR outperforms existing method. The images with and without image enhancement scheme produce a huge difference in the results.

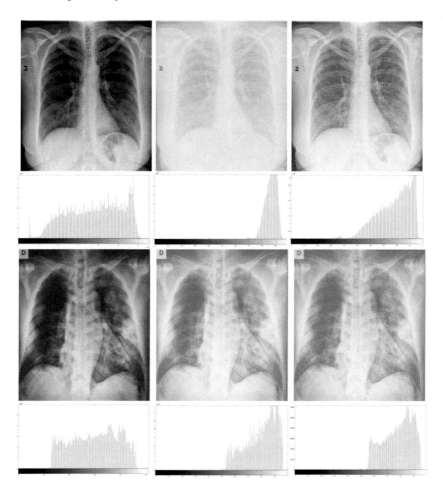

Fig. 1 (continued)

Table 1 Performance comparison based on PSNR, CEP, and LEP

Test images	MSRCR			Proposed improved MSRCR		
	PSNR	CEP	LEP	PSNR	CEP	LEP
1.	36.77	0.118	**0.132**	**36.95**	**0.133**	0.131
2.	**32.83**	**0.172**	0.167	32.82	0.171	**0.177**
3.	35.90	0.397	**0.174**	**35.94**	**0.399**	0.173
4.	34.34	0.134	0.128	**34.36**	**0.141**	**0.134**

Table 2 Performance comparison on approximate and detailed wavelet energy

Test images	Org. image		MSRCR		Proposed improved MSRCR	
	Approx.	Detail	Approx.	Detail	Approx.	Detail
1.	99.34	0.339	99.50	0.327	**99.57**	**0.409**
2.	99.62	0.252	**99.69**	0.302	99.59	**0.392**
3.	99.41	0.387	99.10	0.390	**99.71**	**0.411**
4.	99.67	0.283	**99.97**	0.112	99.81	**0.390**

This is evident from the experimental result presented. With the image enhancement algorithm applied, the visual details are visible to the naked eye. The doctors can locate any abnormalities by verifying each corner of the cells. The proposed image enhancement scheme is a big boon to the doctors, radiologists, and researchers in making right decisions to identify COVID-19 cases.

References

1. Hosseiny, M., Kooraki, S., Gholamrezanezhad, A., Reddy, S., & Myers, L. (2020). Radiology perspective of coronavirus disease 2019 (COVID-19): Lessons from severe acute respiratory syndrome and middle east respiratory syndrome. *American Journal of Roentgenology AJR, 214,* 1–5.
2. Mukherjee, H., Ghosh, S., Dhar, A., Obaidullah, S. K. M., Santosh, K. C., & Roy, K. Shallow convolutional neural network for COVID-19 outbreak screening using chest X-rays. https://doi.org/10.36227/techrxiv.12156522.v1.
3. Chung, M., Bernheim, A., Mei, X., et al. (4 February 2020). CT imaging features of 2019 novel coronavirus (2019-nCoV). *Radiology* (In Press).
4. Fernandes, S. L., Rajinikanth, V., & Kadry, S. (2019). A hybrid framework to evaluate breast abnormality using infrared thermal images. *IEEE Consumer Electronics Magazine, 8*(5), 31–36. https://doi.org/10.1109/MCE.2019.2923926.
5. Gomez, P., Semmler, M., Schutzenberger, A., Bohr, C., & Dollinger, M. (2019). Low-light image enhancement of high-speed endoscopic videos using a convolutional neural network. *Medical and Biological Engineering and Computing, 57*(7), 1451–1463.
6. https://www.who.int/emergencies/diseases/novel-coronavirus-2019/global-research-on-novel-coronavirus-2019-ncov.
7. Hashemi, S., Kiani, S., Noroozi, N., & Moghaddam, M. E. (2010). An image contrast enhancement method based on genetic algorithm. *Pattern Recognition Letter, 31*(13), 1816–1824.
8. Hanumantharaju, M. C., Manjunath Aradhya, V. N., Ravishankar, M., & Mamatha, A. (2012). A particle swarm optimization method for tuning the parameters of multiscale retinex based color image enhancement. In *Proceedings of the International Conference on Advances in Computing, Communications and Informatics,* pp. 721–727.
9. Zhang, R., Huang, Y., & Zhen, Z. (2011). A ultrasound liver image enhancement algorithm based on multi-scale Retinex theory. In *5th International Conference on Bioinformatics and Biomedical Engineering, (ICBBE),* pp. 1–3.
10. Dey, N., et al. (2019). Social-group-optimization based tumor evaluation tool for clinical brain MRI of Flair/diffusion-weighted modality. *Biocybernetics and Biomedical Engineering, 39*(3), 843–856. https://doi.org/10.1016/j.bbe.2019.07.005.

11. Satapathy, S. C., Raja, N. S. M., Rajinikanth, V., Ashour, A. S., & Dey, N. (2018). Multi-level image thresholding using Otsu and chaotic bat algorithm. *Neural Computing and Applications, 29*(12), 1285–1307. https://doi.org/10.1007/s00521-016-2645-5.
12. Rundo, L., Tangherloni, A., Nobile, M., Militello, C., Besozzi, D., Mauri, G., et al. (2019). MedGA: A novel evolutionary method for image enhancement in medical imaging systems. *Expert Systems with Applications, 119,* 387–399.
13. Jobson, D. J., Rahman, Z., & Woodell, G. A. (1997). Properties and performance of a center/surround retinex. *IEEE Transactions on Image Processing, 6*(3), 451–462.
14. Hanumantharaju, M. C., Ravishankar, M., Rameshbabu, D. R., & Aradhya, M. (2014). A new framework for Retinex-based colour image enhancement using particle swarm optimization. *International Journal of Swarm Intelligence, 1*(2), 133–155.
15. Setty, S., Srinath, N., & Hanumantharaju, M. (2013). Development of multiscale Retinex algorithm for medical image enhancement based on multi-rate sampling. In *Proceedings of International conference on Signal Processing, Image Processing and Pattern Recognition (ICSIPR)*, pp. 1–6.
16. Hanumantharaju, M. C., Ravishankar, M., & Rameshbabu, D. R. (2014). Natural color image enhancement based on modified multiscale Retinex algorithm and performance evaluation using wavelet energy. In *Recent Advances in Intelligent Informatics. Advances in Intelligent Systems and Computing*, vol. 235. Springer.
17. Shen, C. T., & Hwang, W. L. (2009). Color image enhancement using Retinex with robust envelop. In *Proceedings of International Conference on Image Processing (ICIP-2009)*.
18. Jobson, D. J., Rahman, Z. U., & Woodell, G. A. (1997). A multiscale retinex for bridging the gap between color images and the human observation of scenes. *IEEE Transactions on Image processing, 6*(7), 965-976.
19. Kimmel, R., Elad, M., Shaked, D., Keshet, R., & Sobel, I. (2003). A variational framework for Retinex. *International Journal on Computer Vision, 52*(1), 7–23.
20. Hanumantharaju, M. C., Ravishankar, M., Babu, D. R. R., & Aradhya, V. N. M. (2011). An efficient metric for evaluating the quality of color image enhancement. In *Indian International Conference on Artificial Intelligence, 2011*, pp. 1016–1026.
21. https://github.com/ieee8023/covid-chestxray-dataset.

Deep Learning-Based COVID-19 Diagnosis and Trend Predictions

Juanying Xie, Mingzhao Wang, and Ran Liu

Abstract During the Chinese Spring Festival travel rush in 2020, a new type of pneumonia disease, named COVID-19 subsequently broke out in Wuhan, Hubei province, China. The COVID-19 was quickly spreading in China and emerged nearly all over the world. In this chapter, our motivation is to adopt the deep learning techniques to help clinic doctors to diagnose the patients of COVID-19 and predict the trend of COVID-19. To realize our motivation, we on the one hand adopt deep learning techniques to analyse CT images of patients. The transfer learning and data augmentation techniques are adopted for the lacking of samples in our obtained CT image data set. We build a model by designing and training a new deep network to help clinic doctors to make an appropriate diagnose decision. On the other hand, according to the spreading characteristics of COVID-19 and the controlling measures adopted by Chinese government, we propose to modify the classic SEIR (susceptible-exposed-infectious-recovered) model and establish a new SEIR dynamics model with considering the infectiousness of the people in the latent period and the quarantine period. The appropriate parameters of our modified SEIR model are learned by using deep learning techniques. Our proposed deep learning-based diagnosis for COVID-19 can help medicine doctors to make an appropriate diagnostic decision. Our modified SEIR model can effectively predict the transmission trend of COVID-19 and can be used for short-term trend prediction of the epidemic.

Keywords COVID-19 · Artificial intelligence · Deep learning · CT images · SEIR model

J. Xie (✉) · R. Liu
School of Computer Science, Shaanxi Normal University, Xi'an 710119, China
e-mail: xiejuany@snnu.edu.cn

R. Liu
e-mail: lroriginal@163.com

M. Wang
College of Life Sciences, Shaanxi Normal University, Xi'an 710119, China
e-mail: wangmz2014@163.com

1   Introduction

It was reported that there was an atypical pneumonia with unknown aetiology appeared in Wuhan, the capital city of Hubei province in China, in December 2019. Subsequently, it was detected that this atypical pneumonia was a new coronavirus [1]. The new coronavirus was first named as 2019 novel coronavirus (2019-nCOV) by World Health Organization (WHO) on January 20, 2020, and the pneumonia caused by it was named as COVID-19 on February 11, 2020 [2]. Patients with COVID-19 generally have symptoms similar to SARS patients, such as cough, fever, dyspnea, acute respiratory syndrome and kidney failure. [3, 4]. In addition, chest computed tomography (CT) images showed that there were diffuse and small ground glass nodules in the bilateral lungs of COVID-19 patients [5]. It is reported that the natural host of 2019-nCOV is likely to be bats [6, 7], but the intermediate host is still unknown [8]. Moreover, the evidence shows that it can lead the infections from person-to-person [9, 10]. Although we do not know where the 2019-nCOV comes from, it is the indisputable fact that the COVID-19 has spreaded to nearly all of the countries in the world and has become a very serious global pandemic. As of April 15, 2020, the accumulative number of infections in the worldwide has exceeded 1.95 million, and the number of deaths is about 130,000. This epidemic has already brought a major impact on the world's public health and the economy of the world.

This 2019-nCOV just happened before the Chinese Spring Festival. The huge personnel flow advanced the spread of it to other regions in China. In order to stop the propagation of the epidemic and minimize its impact on the public health and the national economy, the Chinese government quickly launched the "Level I response to major public health emergencies", and ordered to block the Wuhan city on January 23, 2020, and cut off all transportations between Wuhan and any other cities in China. Meanwhile, China government called on all of Chinese to stay at home, and wearing masks when he/she must leave home to go to public places, and suspending some intra-city public transportations, closing entertainment venues and banning public gatherings, so as to block the spreading of this serious infectious disease COVID-19. In addition, there are many artificial intelligence (AI) experts devoted themselves to do related researches about COVID-19, published or issued many related papers. Although the situations in China were much better after two months, the COVID-19 was still serious in many other countries. The medicine doctors are not enough compared to the rising up COVID-19 patients. So, it needs us, all of AI researchers, to use AI technologies to do some work about the COVID-19, and to help humankind to overcome the crisis.

In this chapter, we will present our two studies about COVID-19. The first is that our doing analysis to the CT images of patients by using deep learning techniques, while using the transfer learning and data augmentation technologies to solve the problem of over-fitting due to the small number of samples in the data set we obtained. We modified the RetinaNet networks, so as to learn the high-level abstract features of CT images of patients. The second is that we present a new modified SEIR dynamics model with considering the infectivity of an individual in latent period and the quarantine period. Those appropriate parameters of the new modified SEIR model are learned by using deep learning techniques. Our motivation is to help clinic doctors make appropriate diagnostic decisions, and help whoever related to make efficient prediction to the short-term trend for the COVID-19 epidemic, so as to provide decision-makers a basis to prevent and control the new infectious disease.

2 Related Work

Deep learning is a branch of machine learning. Its aim lies in establishing while simulating the human brain neural networks to do analysis and learn. It imitates the ways of human brains to analyse images, sounds, texts and various kinds of data. The essential of deep learning is artificial deep neural network, and its structure is a multi-layer perceptron with multi-hidden layers. The advantages of deep learning are that it can automatically extract features and get a high-level abstract representation of the data. It has been used in many fields, including early screening and diagnosis of medical images [11].

Due to the strengths of deep learning, it is believed by researchers that this technology will play invaluable roles in controlling and help diagnose COVID-19. Therefore, many researchers have used deep learning to study COVID-19, so as to help humankind to overcome the crisis. The deep learning-based model for detecting COVID-19 using the high-resolution computed tomography was published by researchers from Wuhan University People's Hospital and Wuhan EndoAngel Medical Technology Company on medRxiv platform [12]. To validate the constructed deep learning model, this study collected and processed 46,096 anonymous CT images of 106 inpatients in Wuhan University People's Hospital. The results showed that the developed deep learning-based model had got a comparable performance to that of radiologists and significantly reduced the work stress of radiologists. A customized deep convolutional neural network was proposed for detecting the COVID-19 cases from chest X-ray (CXR) images by the researchers from the University of Waterloo [13]. The findings of this study showed that the potent promising results could be achieved in detecting COVID-19 with chest radiographs. Mukherjee et al. [14] proposed a lightweight convolutional neural network (CNN)-tailored shallow architecture to detect COVID-19 positive cases using chest X-rays automatically from non-COVID ones. They obtained the accuracy of 96.92%, sensitivity of 0.942 and AUC of 0.9869 by using 260 chest X-rays, and the false positive rate was 0 for 130 COVID-19 positive cases. Considering the CXR images can be obtained easier than CT images. Das et al. [15] proposed a deep learning-based CNN model to filter COVID-19 positive CXRs from non-COVID ones. They concluded that they achieved the best results among the existing AI-driven tools in detecting out COVID-19 by using CXRs. Rajinikanth et al. [16] proposed an image-assisted system to extract COVID-19 infected sections from lung CT images, so as to assist clinic doctors to detect out COVID-19 patients and help to plan an appropriate treatment process.

The SEIR model is a common disease transmission dynamics model [17]. Since SEIR model takes the latent into account compared to the SIR model, it has been applied to the analysis and prediction of many major infectious diseases, such as severe acute respiratory syndrome (SARS) [18] and Middle East respiratory syndrome (MERS) [19] and human immunodeficiency virus (HIV) [20]. At present, the SEIR model is also used by many researchers in predicting and analysing the development trend of the COVID-19 epidemic. Based on the transmission characteristics of 2019-nCOV, Tang et al. [21] brought forward the deterministic SEIR compartmental transmission dynamics model with a comprehensive consideration of the clinical progression, close contact and isolation of the disease and other interventions, and predicted that the epidemic peak would be around February 5. Cao et al. [22] incorporated the characteristics of COVID-19 incubation patients with infectious ability into the SEIR model and proposed a modified SEIR dynamics model that jointly took the infectivity of the individuals in the incubation period and the influence from the isolation intervention into account. This modified SEIR model parameters were solved by using the Euler integral method. As a result, it can effectively simulate and forecast the development of the epidemic situation of Hubei province. Yang et al. [23] integrated population migration data and COVID-19 epidemiological data into the SEIR model to forecast the development trend of COVID-19, and they also used the SARS data in 2003 to train a long short-term memory (LSTM) model to forecast the number of new infections.

3 Deep Learning for COVID-19 Diagnosis

From the aforementioned studies in Sect. 2, we can see that deep learning techniques have been adopted to detect the COVID-19 patients by learning the CT images. Compared with reverse transcription polymerase chain reaction (RT-PCR) detection method, the deep learning-based CT image examination is timely, accurate, and with high positive rate. Furthermore, the range of lung lesions is closely related to clinical symptoms. Therefore, the CT image-based diagnosis is a preferring one for diagnosing COVID-19. It was reported that the most important way to make the accurate diagnosis is to read CT images for clinic doctors during COVID-19 epidemic in China, and the decisions by analysing the CT images were with high positive rate. For patients' CT images, a deep learning model aims to learn the abstract mapping between the raw data and the expected clinical outcomes. If there are enough samples, after many training iterations, the expected output of the final model will infinitely approximate the real labels. We show the working process of the deep learning techniques in Fig. 1.

On account of the privacy protection, CT images of patients are not always open and accessed freely. Even though the current COVID-CT data set is open, the number of samples contained in the data set is insignificant, and it is still difficult to achieve the amount of data required by the deep learning model. This greatly impedes the accuracy of detecting COVID-19 patients by the CT images using deep learning

Fig. 1 Schematic workflow of a deep learning model

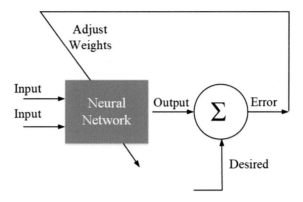

techniques. Because training deep learning model on such a small data set is very easy to fall into over-fitting, which makes the model perform well on the training data, but bad on the test data, such that the generalization performance of model is poor. In addition, there are no existing principles for designing network structures for specific tasks. Fortunately, there are three solutions to these aforementioned problems:

I.   It is well-known that transfer learning is the most commonly used method in deep learning which uses large amounts of data from related fields to assist model training and learning. For example, a large number of CXR images can be used to pretrain a deep convolutional neural network, and then fine-tune the trained network on the COVID-CT data set, which can achieve twice the result with half the effort.

II. Create new images from limited training data and add them to the original training set. The methods to create new images include expanding the original images by flipping, rotating and translating. This method is called data augmentation and is the most common technique in deep learning to solve over-fitting problems caused by the lacking of training data.

III. Combine the above two methods. That is, use the augmented data to fine-tune the pretrain model.

4   Prediction Model About COVID-19 Outbreak

The SEIR epidemic model is a classic disease transmission model based on complex networks. It has been used to model and analyse the infectious diseases such as SARS, MERS and HIV. The SEIR model classifies people into four categories: susceptible (S), exposed (E), infectious (I) and recovered (R). Figure 2 displays the processes to establish the classic SEIR model.

Considering the quarantine measures taken by the Chinese government for preventing and controlling COVID-19, we added the quarantined susceptible (S_q) and the quarantined exposed (E_q) categories to the classic SEIR model. The quarantined individuals are divided into S_q and E_q according to whether they are infected

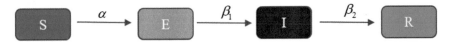

Fig. 2 Classic SEIR epidemic dynamics model, where α is the infection probability of the susceptible, β_1 is the probability of the exposed being transformed into the infected and β_2 is the recovery
probability

or not. The quarantined susceptible ones become the susceptible (S) again after
being released and the quarantined exposed ones become exposed (E) category after
releasing quarantine if they do not show symptoms of infection during the quarantine period. In addition, we consider that the exposed individuals also have got the
ability to infect the virus to the susceptible individuals. Our modified SEIR epidemic
dynamic model is shown in Fig. 3, where α_1 is the infection probability of the
susceptible by the infected, and α_2 is the infection probability of the susceptible by
the exposed. The appropriate parameters of our modified SEIR model are obtained
using deep learning techniques.

We proposed a two-stage SEIR model to forecast this COVID-19 prevalence in
Shaanxi province before and after the response to the "level I response to major
public health emergencies" on January 25, 2020. In the first stage, due to insuffi-
cient knowledge about COVID-19, Shaanxi province did not take any prevention
and control measures against COVID-19 before January 25, 2020. So, we use the
classic SEIR model to make the prediction for this COVID-19 development trend.
In the second phase, after January 25, 2020, Shaanxi province implemented various
measures such as restricted travel, wearing masks and isolating contacts. Therefore,
we adopted the revised SEIR model to predict the COVID-19 epidemic situation
for this stage. Meanwhile, we also calculated the basic reproduction number of two
stages by changing the value of the parameters to simulate the development trend of
COVID-19 infection before and after taking prevention and control measures. The
study results show that the measures such as home prevention and control quarantine
and centralized treatment taken by Chinese government have greatly suppressed the
widespread spread of the COVID-19 epidemic, and also gained valuable time and
reference for other countries to control the COVID-19 epidemic.

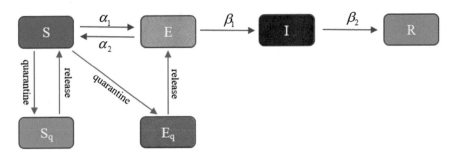

Fig. 3 Our proposed SEIR epidemic dynamics model to simulate COVID-19

5 Conclusions

In our study about COVID-19, we first adopt the deep learning methods to analyse and identify the COVID-19 patients by CT images, where we combined the transfer learning and data augmentation technologies to solve the over-fitting problem due to the small size of data set. The deep learning-based COVID-19 studies can help medicine doctors quickly obtain diagnostic results and make appropriate decisions in a short time. Then taking into account the transmission characteristics of 2019-nCOV virus and the epidemic prevention measures in China, we established a new modified SEIR epidemic dynamics model. A two-stage SEIR epidemic dynamics model was proposed based on this new model to analyse the transmission pattern of COVID-19 in Shaanxi province. The appropriate parameters for our two-stage SEIR epidemic model are learned by using the deep learning technologies. Our destination is to help humankind to overcome the COVID-19 pandemic crisis. We hope that our study could help clinic doctors to make the correct diagnosis to the patients of COVID-19 as fast as possible and provide some references about prevention and control measures for other countries in the world.

Acknowledgements This work is supported by the NSFC under Grant No. 61673251, and by the NKRDPC under Grant No. 2016YFC0901900, and by the Fundamental Research Funds for the Central Universities under Grant No. GK201806013, and by the Innovation Funds for Graduate Programs in Shaanxi Normal University under Grant Nos. 2016CSY009 and 2018TS078.

References

1. Li, Q., Guan, X., & Wu, P. (2020). Early transmission dynamics in Wuhan, China, of novel coronavirus–infected pneumonia. *New England Journal of Medicine*.
2. Xinhuanet.com (2020) WHO named the novel coronavirus pneumonia as COVID-19. Available from: http://www.xinhuanet.com/world/2020-02/12/c_1125561389.htm.
3. Chen, Nanshan, Zhou, Min, & Dong, Xuan. (2020). Epidemiological and clinical characteristics of 99 cases of 2019 novel coronavirus pneumonia in Wuhan, China: a descriptive study. *The Lancet, 395*(10223), 507–513.
4. Guan, W., Ni, Z., & Hu, Y. (2020). Clinical characteristics of 2019 novel coronavirus infection in China. *MedRxiv*.
5. Qu, J., Yang, R., Song, L., & Kamel, I. R. (2020). Atypical lung feature on chest CT in a lung adenocarcinoma cancer patient infected with COVID-19. *Annals of Oncology*.
6. Xu, X., Chen, P., & Wang, J. (2020). Evolution of the novel corona-virus from the ongoing Wuhan outbreak and modeling of its spike protein for risk of human transmission. *Science China-life Sciences, 63*(3), 457–460.
7. Zhou, P., Yang, X., & Wang, X. (2020). A pneumonia outbreak associated with a new coronavirus of probable bat origin. *Nature, 579*(7798), 270–273.
8. Cyranoski, David. (2020). Mystery deepens over animal source of coronavirus. *Nature, 579*(7797), 18–19.
9. Chan, J. F. W., Yuan, S., & Kok, K. H. (2020). A familial cluster of pneumonia associated with the 2019 novel coronavirus indicating person-to-person transmission: a study of a family cluster. *The Lancet, 395*(10223), 514–523.

10. Rothe, C., Schunk, M., & Sothmann, P. (2020). Transmission of 2019-nCoV infection from an asymptomatic contact in Germany. *New England Journal of Medicine, 382*(10), 970–971.
11. Xie, J., Liu, R., Luttrell IV, J., & Zhang, C. (2019). Deep learning based analysis of histopathological images of breast cancer. *Frontiers in Genetics, 10,* 80.
12. Chen, J., Wu, L., & Zhang, J. (2020). Deep learning-based model for detecting 2019 novel coronavirus pneumonia on high-resolution computed tomography: A prospective study. *MedRxi.*
13. Wang, L., & Wong, A. (2020). COVID-Net: A tailored deep convolutional neural network design for detection of COVID-19 cases from chest radiography images. *ArXiv preprint* arXiv: 2003.09871.
14. Mukherjee, H., Ghosh, S., Dhar, A., Obaidullah, M. S., Santosh, K. C., & Roy, K. (2020). Shallow convolutional neural network for COVID-19 outbreak screening using chest X-rays. *Techrxiv, 12156522,* v1.
15. Das, D., Santosh, K. C., & Pal, U. (2020). Truncated inception net: COVID-19 outbreak screening using chest X-rays. *Research Square.* https://doi.org/10.21203/rs.3.rs-20795/v1.
16. Rajinikanth, V., Dey, N., Raj, A. N. J., Hassanien, A. E., Santosh, K. C., & Raja, N. S. R. (2020). Harmony-search and Otsu based system for coronavirus disease (COVID-19) detection using lung CT scan images. *ArXiv preprint* arXiv:2004.03431.
17. Miller, W. (2002). *Mathematical approaches for emerging and reemerging infectious diseases: Models, methods, and theory.* New York, NY: Springer.
18. Dye, C., & Gay, N. (2003). Modeling the SARS epidemic. *Science, 300*(5627), 1884–1885.
19. Eifan, S. A., Nour, I., & Hanif, A. (2017). A pandemic risk assessment of Middle East respiratory syndrome coronavirus (MERS-CoV) in Saudi Arabia. *Saudi Journal of Biological Sciences, 24*(7), 1631–1638.
20. Zakary, O., Elmouki, I., & Rachik, M. (2016). On the impact of awareness programs in HIV/AIDS prevention: An SIR model with optimal control. *International Journal of Computer Applications, 133*(9), 1–6.
21. Tang, B., Wang, X., & Li, Q. (2020). Estimation of the transmission risk of the 2019-nCoV and its implication for public health interventions. *Journal of Clinical Medicine, 9*(2), 462.
22. Cao, S., Feng, P., Shi, P. (2020). Study on the epidemic development of corona virus disease-19 (COVID-19) in Hubei province by a modified SEIR model, *Journal of Zhejiang University, 49*(2):178–184.
23. Yang, Z., Zeng, Z., Wang, K., Wong, S. S., Liang, W., Zanin, M. et al. (2020). Modified SEIR and AI prediction of the epidemics trend of COVID-19 in China under public health interventions. *Journal of Thoracic Disease, 12*(3):165–174.

COVID-19: Loose Ends

Minakshi Pradeep Atre

Abstract The sudden outburst of the COVID-19 has hit the world badly. Avoid, control, and monitor (ACM) is the need of time! With limited expert manpower in COVID-19, the technologies like artificial intelligence (AI), robotics (R), and IOT (I), i.e., (ARI) would help in avoidance of further spread and control of disease transmission. Prediction and analysis tools are effectively implemented only when sufficient data is available. Though an early stage of any pandemic has to deal with the scarcity of data, an early detection and prediction are equally important steps to fight COVID-19. But a complete solution to the pandemic is impossible because of the loose ends like availability of data and "dependent" development of ARI technology. Since December 2019, there has been a continuous up-scaling in analysis and prediction algorithms because of more data getting available in terms of features and more number of the cases across the world. This chapter will discuss the role of ARI and loose ends in their implementation. It is focused on three major aspects: AI algorithms in analysis and prediction, the use of robotics in control and prevention of the pandemic and the role of IOT for the patient monitoring system (PMS). This discussion will provide an evolutionary path of the algorithms. The accuracy rate for diagnosis and prediction has been increased because of the various novel approaches by researchers. They are trying to overcome the loopholes and are tying the loose ends with the advent of more and more data!

Keywords COVID-19 · AI · IOT · Robotics · Avoid-Control-Monitor (ACM) · Loose ends · Patient monitoring systems (PMS)

1 Introduction

The outbreak of COVID-19 (**CO**rona **VI**rus **D**isease-2019) happened first in Wuhan, China in December 2019 [12] and then rapidly spread across the world. This was later named as nCov, an abbreviation for "novel Corona." The scientists have not

M. P. Atre (✉)
Department of E&TC, PVG's COET, Pune, SPPU, Pune, India
e-mail: mpatre29@gmail.com

© The Author(s), under exclusive license to Springer Nature Singapore Pte Ltd. 2020
A. Joshi et al. (eds.), *Intelligent Systems and Methods to Combat Covid-19*,
SpringerBriefs in Computational Intelligence,
https://doi.org/10.1007/978-981-15-6572-4_8

developed any vaccinations till date, though they could find the reason immediately. To deal with such a pandemic, often a teamwork of the scientists, technologists, engineers, and mathematicians is needed. The technology is growing fast and helping the life sciences to avoid, control, and monitor such diseases. The AI or machine learning algorithms can be exploited to predict and gain control over this pandemic. The algorithms would help to understand and model the spread factor of the nCov beforehand and analyze the case fatality ratio (CFR) [1, 2], based on different COVID-19 parameters.

As said earlier, a complete IOT-based system or an AI algorithm cannot be developed unless the loose ends are tied up. The first limitation is **data:** the larger datasets would help in more accurate detection and prediction of the pandemic. The standards and protocols must be defined for the exchange of patients' data, respecting the privacy of a patient. The second limitation is **benchmark datasets and clinical study** [7]. COVID-19 is novel coronavirus and being in early stage there is no benchmark dataset available. The other aspect is the completely dynamic nature of the disease. It changes quickly from time to time, person to person, culture to culture, and place to place [8]. The third limitation is **accessing the information through IOT devices for patient monitoring systems (PMS).** It includes the mobile phones and wearable devices like smart watches. There is a need for standardization of protocols to encourage communication between devices and across systems without compromising data safety and preventing data oversight [11]. These three main loose ends could be addressed with one question unanswered, what would happen if there is second transmission cycle? Because all the analysis techniques have one underlying assumption of no second cycle of COVID-19 transmission.

This chapter is divided into three sections. Section 2 discusses the parameters of COVID-19 while Sect. 3 discusses the modeling techniques for different phases of COVID-19 and loose ends in modeling techniques. And Sect. 4 illustrates the role of artificial intelligence (AI) and Internet of things (IoT) in patient monitoring system.

2 Discussion of Parameters of COVID-19

There are three aspects of COVID-19 parameters. The first is the set of person dependent parameters, the second is the set of global parameters, and the third is COVID-19 symptoms. The symptoms would depend on these two parameters. The person dependent parameters will include diet, age, vaccinations, travel history, and medical history (prevailing diseases like blood pressure, diabetes, asthma). The chapter enlists the symptoms as: loss of smell (major), with other symptoms as, fatigue, fever, cough, diarrhea, and shortness of breath [4]. The global parameters would include geographical location, atmospheric temperature, and miscellaneous parameters (like few people believed health getting affected by 5G). Figure 1 depicts the parameters and symptoms of COVID-19.

Figure 2 shows the number of nCov cases exhibiting the combinational symptoms. This reference paper claims that the very first dominant symptom is loss of smell. The

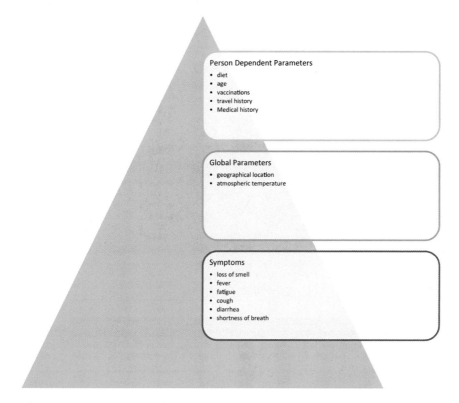

Fig. 1 COVID-19: key aspects

reference says diarrhea and shortness of breath appear later than the loss of smell. The challenge is to identify how fast the symptoms develop and is there a particular sequence of these symptoms. The modeling techniques completely depend on such critical parameters. The phases of disease will be identified depending on the % value of these symptoms. The critical phase includes the pneumonia infection in the lungs.

3 Modeling Techniques for Different Phases of COVID-19

Figure 3 depicts the phases of this pandemic. It is divided into different phases: symptomatic phase [3], confirmation phase after the incubation period, medication phase and recovery period for the COVID-19.

A model can be developed for the symptomatic and incubation phases once the COVID-19 symptoms are identified for variety of patients. Sources like WHO, NHS(UK), and other governmental medical organizations could be used to obtain

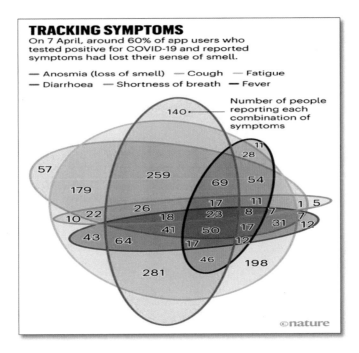

Fig. 2 Tracking symptoms *Source* COVID symptom tracker team, UK

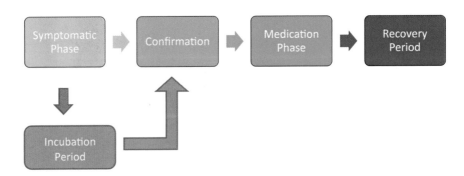

Fig. 3 Depiction of the phases of corona (COVID-19)

the data required for the fast and accurate implementation of the models. The symptomatic phase along with the incubation period is modeled by Stephen Lauer et al. [3] by using log-normal distribution. They estimated the mean incubation period for the collected database of 181 cases. They also tried to overcome the possible bias on the result by the patients with normal cough and fever symptoms. The incubation period estimation is also verified with other parametric distributions like Weibull, Gamma, and Erlang distributions. What affects these results are (1) the correct discrimination of normal cough and fever patients from nCov patients and (2) the exact onset time for incubation estimation! Algorithms can be developed to distinguish the normal and nCov coughs. The loose ends, that need to tied up!!

There are two categories of the confirmation of COVID-19: local and global. A local confirmation is the confirmation of the COVID-19 patient's stage of health while the global confirmation can be done on the large scale, i.e., the phase of the spread of the epidemic which counts the number of patients per country. Phase-1, phase-2, phase-3, phase-4, and phase-5 are the global stages of this epidemic [2]. An exponential graph depicts the phase of the epidemic. A country-wise count is the global confirmed number of cases. For the correct local and global COVID-19 confirmation, the data must be regularly and immediately updated. This contributes to the spread factor analysis of COVID-19 and the graph plotting of virus transmission. Data (number of patients) updating on global level seems to be a limitation!

The confirmation phase has been implemented by using various AI-driven tools. It is modeled using one of the predictive analysis techniques like decision tree techniques in [10]. This was also used previously in prediction of SARS epidemic. The researchers implemented decision tree with gain ratio and Gini index for the prediction analysis. The proposed work by authors in [7] aims to extract and evaluate the coronavirus (COVID-19) caused pneumonia infection in lung using CT scans. An image-assisted system will be implemented to extract COVID-19 infected sections from lung CT scans with the final expected view, named as "coronal view."

After the confirmation phase, medication phase is the most challenging phase at this point of time where the doctors are using combinational medicines for the recovery. With sudden arrival and rapid spread of COVID-19, the death rate was really high. The researchers were trying to analyze the COVID-19 transmission graph. The global data was expressed with the term "case fatality ratio (CFR)." It is calculated by dividing the number of known deaths by the number of known cases [1]. The loophole was the accuracy to identify the nCov cases. The spread factor was not possible to be calculated because of the complex dependency of the symptomatic phase. It has dependency on many parameters as: how the virus is transmitted, how much is the incubation period, had the infected come in contact with others, and the most important, the reproductive number R0 of the virus [2]. (The ongoing research on coronavirus has not confirmed with R0 parameter.) These are the loose ends, need to tie up.

The last phase of recovery has again complex dependency but similar to confirmation phase modeling, a binary tree will be helpful with sufficient amount of data. Figure 4 below summarizes the modeling techniques for the different phases of the COVID-19.

Apart from the analysis and prediction of COVID-19 at different phases, the transmission of disease also needs to be modeled and a transmission structure needs to be developed as a precautionary measure. The researchers [9] used **auto-encoders with latent variables** and clustering algorithms to group the provinces for investigating the transmission across that province. Another novel forecasting model has been developed in an early phase of COVID-19 **despite the limited data** by the researchers in the article [5]. A polynomial neural network with corrective feedback (PNN + cf) was developed for the forecasting of COVID-19 transmission.

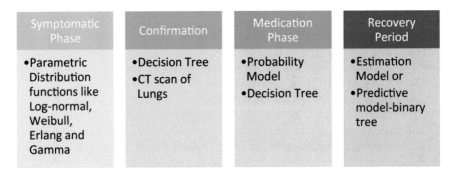

Symptomatic Phase	Confirmation	Medication Phase	Recovery Period
•Parametric Distribution functions like Log-normal, Weibull, Erlang and Gamma	•Decision Tree •CT scan of Lungs	•Probability Model •Decision Tree	•Estimation Model or •Predictive model-binary tree

Fig. 4 Deploying the COVID-19 model

The authors in [6] state that "Considering the spread rate of COVID-19 across the globe, AI-driven tools are expected to work as cross-population train/test models." The researchers in the article [8] also used Composite Monte-Carlo (CMC) approach toward forecasting of COVID-19 under high uncertainty by **extrapolating the available data**. The researchers in the above articles have used different AI-driven tools to overcome the scarcity of the data with one **underlying assumption of no second transmission.**

4 Role of AI, Robotics, and IOT

An insight into the symptoms of COVID-19 and the loose ends in the modeling process have been discussed in previous two sections. This section discusses how, the three major areas of technology, AI, IOT, robotics can be exploited in the entire process of ACM.

The different phases of the COVID-19 could be modeled successfully by tying up the loose ends mentioned earlier, by using the artificial intelligence or machine learning algorithms. Calculation of spread factor, the probability of infection, the estimation of recovery could be solved using machine learning algorithms. The most important factor to track the travel history of the person is through his mobile GPS and use it to estimate the spread factor.

As discussed in Sect. 3, AI algorithms (models) can be categorized as: **prediction model** to estimate the number of patients and if the person is at the risk of COVID-19 in incubation period, and **recovery model** to estimate the chances of survival.

By modeling the features of the COVID-19, the control mechanisms can be further developed using drones, the robotics.

The drones could be used for (1) spraying disinfectants, (2) surveillance, i.e., detection of mobility and movement of people and alert message to control room, wait for further instructions, and spray disinfectant/hit and alarm, (3) identification of cluster and intimation to control room. A fully equipped drone system can be designed to control and avoid the spread of COVID-19. The three pillars of science and technology to win over COVID-19:

AI: for prediction modeling

Robotics: sanitization drones as precautionary measures.

IOT: IOT-based systems for monitoring the quarantined persons.

Internet of things is another major technology which can be deployed on two major fronts, first in **isolation homes on individual scale** and the second front is on large scale **for monitoring and tracking of quarantined** person.

In isolation homes, IOT can be used for:

(1) maintaining the optimum room temperature for speedy recovery (using ACs and radiators)
(2) keeping the spirits of the patient high by playing upbeat music, encouraging audiobooks and suggesting inspiring movies
(3) keeping the patient updated about COVID-19
(4) ensuring the patient follows hygiene etiquette
(5) reminding him/her about taking medications, if any
(6) providing excellent communication facilities to make sure he can talk to his friends, relatives, etc.

The second front tasks majorly include

(1) Monitoring quarantine people (2) location tracking of a quarantined person, and (3) sending an alert message to local authority if he crosses the boundary. The second task is of utmost importance because of scarcity of space for keeping the quarantined people. In such cases, they can be monitored and tracked silently. And if they disobey by crossing the pre-defined boundary, an alert message can be sent to local authority or control room.

To illustrate the role of AI and IOT, a patient monitoring system (PMS) is proposed here in Fig. 5. It presents the conceptual block schematic of the PMS with all the facilities required for controlling and curing the COVID-19. Further, the parameters discussed in Sect. 1.2 can also be monitored using different sensors. The frequency of monitoring can be selected to be every 2 h or more frequently depending on the stage of COVID-19.

The use of IoT devices reminds the author of this chapter about the suggestions given in the article, [11]. The author strongly feels that an increased data sharing practice must be enforced in the urban health sector while abiding to the dimensions of privacy and security due to the sensitive nature of information. A smart city initiative has been taken up by many countries, and based on this, artificial intelligence with wearable IOT devices can help to trace and track the quarantined person or a patient.

Maintain room
temperature

Reminder of
medicines

Ensuring Hygiene
etiquettes

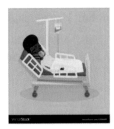

News update regarding
COVID-19

Facility of
Communication
with relatives

Facility of Audio
Books

Playing soothing
music

Fig. 5 Conceptual block schematic of the patient monitoring system

5 Summary

COVID-19 has caused huge damage to the society in terms of number of casualties and economic activity. In order to minimize its effects, an efficient use of science and modern technology such as AI, ML, and IOT must be employed in tandem. The chapter summarizes the loose ends that the scientific and technological community need to address further. It highlights the role of AI-ML algorithms and use of IOT systems in combating the ongoing deadly pandemic. The automation in diagnosis is the need of time because of limited medical experts and that is possible because of ARI technologies. The implementation of PMS system proposed here will ensure quicker control with minimal use of manpower to counter COVID-19.

Acknowledgements I would like to thank my family members, Aditya and Pradeep, for their valuable inputs while writing this chapter.

References

1. Ghani, A. C., et al. (2005). Methods for estimating the case fatality ratio for a novel, emerging infectious disease. *American Journal of Epidemiology, 162*(5), 479–486.
2. Battegay, M., et al. (2020). 2019-novel Coronavirus (2019-nCoV): Estimating the case fatality rate–a word of caution. *Swiss Medical Weekly, 150*, 0506.

3. Lauer, S. A., et al. (2020). The incubation period of coronavirus disease 2019 (COVID-19) from publicly reported confirmed cases: estimation and application. *Annals of Internal Medicine, 172*(9), 577–582.
4. Mayor, S. (2020). Covid-19: Researchers launch app to track spread of symptoms in the UK.
5. Fong, S. J., Li, G., Dey, N., Crespo, R. G., & Herrera-Viedma, E. (2020). Finding an accurate early forecasting model from small dataset: A case of 2019-ncov novel coronavirus outbreak. *arXiv preprint* arXiv:2003.10776.
6. Santosh, K. C. (2020). AI-driven tools for coronavirus outbreak: need of active learning and cross-population train/test models on multitudinal/multimodal data. *Journal of Medical Systems, 44*(5), 1–5.
7. Rajinikanth, V., Dey, N., Raj, A. N. J., Hassanien, A. E., Santosh, K. C., & Raja, N. (2020). Harmony-Search and Otsu based System for Coronavirus Disease (COVID-19) Detection using Lung CT Scan Images. *arXiv preprint* arXiv:2004.03431.
8. Fong, S. J., Li, G., Dey, N., Crespo, R. G., & Herrera-Viedma, E. (2020). Composite Monte Carlo decision making under high uncertainty of novel coronavirus epidemic using hybridized deep learning and fuzzy rule induction. *Applied Soft Computing*, 106282.
9. Hu, Z., Ge, Q., Jin, L., & Xiong, M. (2020). Artificial intelligence forecasting of covid-19 in china. *arXiv preprint* arXiv:2002.07112.
10. Jiang, X., Coffee, M., Bari, A., Wang, J., Jiang, X., Huang, J., … & Wu, Z. (2020). Towards an artificial intelligence framework for data-driven prediction of coronavirus clinical severity. *CMC-Computers, Materials and Continua, 63*(1), 537–551.
11. Allam, Z., Dey, G., & Jones, D. S. (2020). Artificial intelligence (AI) provided early detection of the coronavirus (COVID-19) in China and will influence future Urban health policy internationally. *AI, 1*(2), 156–165.
12. www.who.int.

Social Distancing and Artificial Intelligence—Understanding the Duality in the Times of COVID-19

Deepti Gupta, Amit Mahajan, and Swati Gupta

Abstract It is a well-established fact that 'the human beings are the social beings.' But many a times in a specific situations or circumstances, human beings are forced to adopt and practice social distancing. With the recent outbreak of the pandemic caused by novel coronavirus (COVID-19), people around the world have been advised by the authorities to practice social distancing. This chapter is a modest attempt to study the impact of artificial intelligence on social distancing. AI has contributed and has helped people in different ways in order to maintain social distance. The current situation as well as the advancement of AI in dealing with it has sociological, economic, political, cultural and environmental consequences on the lives of the people all over the world. The present chapter attempts to study the impact of artificial intelligence on maintaining social distancing. The data for understanding the impact on the lives of people shall be collected from the secondary sources as collection of primary data is not possible in this time of coronavirus. The analysis has been done through different case studies related to various technologies which with the help of AI aid in facilitating social distancing and in turn curbing the menace of coronavirus.

Keywords Social distancing · Artificial intelligence · COVID-19 · Community · Technology

D. Gupta (✉)
Department of Sociology, Government MAM College, Cluster University of Jammu, B.R. Ambedkar Road, Jammu 180001, India
e-mail: deepti.ju@gmail.com

A. Mahajan
Centre for IT Enabled Services and Management, University of Jammu, B.R. Ambedkar Road, 180001 Jammu, India
e-mail: amit.mahajans@gmail.com

S. Gupta
Directorate of School Education, Government of Jammu and Kashmir, Jammu 180005, India
e-mail: swatignet@gmail.com

© The Author(s), under exclusive license to Springer Nature Singapore Pte Ltd. 2020
A. Joshi et al. (eds.), *Intelligent Systems and Methods to Combat Covid-19*,
SpringerBriefs in Computational Intelligence,
https://doi.org/10.1007/978-981-15-6572-4_9

1 Introduction

The beginning of the New Year 2020 started with the news about the spread of a cluster of mysterious, suspected pneumonia cases in China with its epicenter in Wuhan, the capital of Hubei province. By the first week of 2020, new coronavirus was identified as the cause of the pneumonia. Since then, it has spread to almost all the countries of the world and has resulted into infecting more than 2.1 million people and leaving at least 142,000 dead. Countries, all over the world are fighting hard to overcome this pandemic.

World Health Organization (WHO) on March 11, 2020 (almost two months after its outbreak) announced the outbreak of coronavirus illness as a pandemic, which had affected more than 118,000 people in over 110 countries and territories around the world and there were chances as well as risk of further spread around the globe [3]. WHO described it as not just public health crises, but a crisis that would touch every sector, so recommended that every individual and every sector should be included in order to fight it. Soon after declaring it a pandemic, WHO, issued certain guidelines to be followed by the people, in order to avoid it from spreading further. One of the major advices was to maintain 'social distancing,' which was rephrased as 'physical distancing' after some time which emphasized the need for physical-not social-distancing from others. This was changed so as to make people remain connected with each other while maintaining physical distances. For the purpose of this chapter phrase 'social distancing' is used, as the physical distances are influencing the social relationships that the people have with each other through the process of face to face verbal and nonverbal interactions.

2 Social Distancing and Its Relevance During the Spread of COVID-19

From the varied experiences of people around the world of this novel coronavirus, it has been concluded that the only available remedy present to the world is social distancing, i.e., avoiding the physical contact with anyone, who can be the probable carrier of this virus. Scientists around the globe are trying hard to device measures to combat this disease which is taking toll on the health system and resulting into number of deaths. Till the medicines or vaccines are designed for this harmful virus, the only measure available for human society is to limit its spread through social distancing.

According to Webster's Dictionary, the word 'social distance' was first used in the year 1824 and was referred to as the level of acceptance or rejection among individuals of different groups. But now after the outbreak of this disease related to coronavirus, social distancing is considered as avoiding a close contact with others so as to prevent the spread of this contagious disease [10]. Social distancing has been enforced in many parts of the world through lockdowns. These enforced lockdowns have slowed down the spread and flattened the curve of this disease. For example, the enforced lockdown by China helped it to curb the spread. China was the first country to put a lockdown into effect in a bid to curb the spread of coronavirus across the nation on January 23, 2020. At that time, the whole world was stunned by the decision taken by China but now after the span of about three months the whole world is under lockdown, i.e., practicing social distancing.

Distancing from the society to protect oneself from getting ill has many problems associated with it. Humans have been the most social of all living beings and our survival depends upon others in the society. Governments are taking all necessary steps to make this lockdown comfortable for the members of the community. If we try to figure out the factors which are responsible for making these lockdowns successful and curbing the spread to the community, then the foremost factor in facilitating this social distancing is the contribution of technology.

3 Artificial Intelligence in the Times of COVID-19

The technologies related to artificial intelligence are considered as the most potential tool which can facilitate the process of defeating this coronavirus pandemic. Artificial intelligence or AI is the use of computer science programming to imitate human thought and action by analyzing data and surroundings, solving or anticipating problems and learning or self-teaching to adapt to a variety of tasks. The term was coined in 1955 by John McCarthy, as 'the science and engineering of making intelligent machines' [9].

Since time, we have witnessed the contribution of AI in different fields of our life. Though the machines have not yet taken over our lives but still they are affecting our lives, our work and our entertainment to the vast extent. There are numerous examples and applications for Artificial intelligence in use today ranging from personal assistants like Alexa and Siri which are voice-powered, to more underlying and fundamental technologies such as behavioral algorithms, suggestive searches and autonomously powered self-driving vehicles boasting powerful predictive capabilities [1].

For the purpose of the present study, AI is understood as machine learning (ML) which is capable of using big data-based models. Natural language processing (NLP), and computer vision application teaches the computers to use this data, which is further processed and used for pattern recognition, explanation, and prediction purposes. For the present study, it has been proved that these functions of the artificial intelligence can be used for the purpose of recognition (diagnose), prediction, and explanation (treatment) of coronavirus infections. The knowledge generated through AI can also be used to manage socio-economic impacts of this pandemic.

4 Impact of AI on Social Distancing

There are many ways through which AI can help in curbing the spread of coronavirus. As we all know that the most efficient way of preventing the spread of this pandemic is social distancing, AI has contributed in developing various tools and technologies which assist the process of social distancing.

Firstly, AI can help in prediction of the spread of these types of viruses. By taking into consideration the data related to the pattern of spread of coronavirus across the world, AI can predict the hotspots. Governments across the nations can use such information to prevent the places becoming hotspots of coronavirus. Thus, the authorities can give early warnings and alerts to people to maintain social distancing and take precautions in those predicted hotspots.

Secondly, AI can help in the detection of the disease by identifying the symptoms. There are various apps being made across nations to identify and detect people with symptom, which in turn can help in curbing the spread of the disease. Those with symptom, detected with the help of AI, can maintain social distance from rest of the community by self-isolating them and can consult the medical professionals if the symptoms become severe. Thus, it also facilitates the process of tracking the contacts or those with symptoms to prevent it from further spread.

Thirdly, AI can facilitate the responses after the disease has been identified. By analyzing the pattern of symptoms and the spread of virus, AI can be used in developing the mode of treatment as well as vaccines and medicines which are most likely to be effective for curing the patients. Machine learning can, thus, result in optimizing the disease management after the outbreak of the disease. The data related to the disease with the help of AI can be used for diagnosis and prognosis purposes. The treatments and cures which are being developed are the outcome of the use of AI tool and technologies.

Lastly, AI can also assist in initiating a response after the outbreak has been contained. It may guide the governments and health agencies to device out a plan to prevent such type of outbreaks in future. Health policies, plans and programs can be initiated by taking into considerations the finding of machine learning. Thus, AI has the potential to assist in the prediction, guidance, controlling the menace of this disease.

There are many success stories whereby, the communities with the help of various applications, which are AI based, have been able to curtail the spread of this infectious virus. In this chapter, the further discussion is on those applications/technologies which are studied as case studies.

5 Case Studies Related to Application of Artificial Intelligence

5.1 Case Study 1

Aarogya Setu Mobile App was launched on April 2, 2020 and was developed by National Informatics Centre. With the help of this application, the Indian government aims to help connect essential health services with the people while India is under lockdown until May 3, 2020. The description of this app is that it is aimed at augmenting the initiatives of the Government of India, particularly the Department of Health, in proactively reaching out to and informing the users of the app regarding risks, best practices and relevant advisories pertaining to the containment of COVID-19.

This mobile application which was launched by the Ministry of Electronics and IT, Government of India, with the objective is to make people aware of coronavirus and COVID-19. This application, which is available in eleven Indian languages including English, uses the location as well as Bluetooth data of the user to notify him/her about the location of the person near them, who is under quarantine or tested positive. It enables people to identify and access their risk of contracting coronavirus infection. It alerts the person if he/she comes in close proximity of, even unknowingly, those who have tested positive for COVID-19. It also includes the detailed information on how to self-isolate in case one develops symptoms and when one needs medical help. Thus, the app calculates the risks and predicts on the basis of people's interaction with others, using Bluetooth technologies, algorithm and artificial intelligence.

5.2 Case Study 2

The success story of Taiwan, a small island in close proximity to China, is another example of the use of AI in combating COVID-19 and curtailing its spread. Early action, centralized command system, frequent-transparent communication, recourse allocation along with integration of big data and technology are the contributing factors in the success of Taiwan.

Taiwan's government combined the data from the National Health Insurance Administration and Immigration Agency and identified 14-day travel history of patients. Along with that, they used the data from citizen's household registration system and foreigner's entry cards to identify individuals, who were at high risk, self-quarantined them and monitored them through their cell phones. This whole data was utilized through artificial intelligence to provide information about patient's travel histories to all the hospitals, clinics, etc. across the country and also to update the people about the hotspots or risky areas which they need to avoid. Thus, AI helped in maintaining social distancing as well as disease prevention.

5.3 *Case Study 3*

Another success story is that of Republic of Korea, who have been able to flatten the curve of spread of coronavirus with the help of using the technologies related to artificial intelligence. They developed the testing kits using AI within weeks of the outbreak. This widespread testing, with the capacity of 15,000 tests per day, targeted the high-risk groups. Smart Quarantine information system was developed using information from Ministry of Justice, the Ministry of Foreign Affairs, airline companies and major telephone telecommunication companies. This information was then processed using AI platforms and then transferred to the medical staff to have full access of the history of the places that the infected person had traveled in the recent past, to identify and isolate or treat them in a timely manner.

Mobile phone technology data was used for self-health check and to receive information regarding precautions, symptoms and the procedure to follow, if the person develops any coronavirus symptom. In order to trace the contacts of an infected person, they processed the data gathered from mobile phones, credit cards transaction records and CCTV footage. This further helped them to publish detailed maps of movements of infected people by using AI.

Artificial intelligence-based tools and technologies were being used and it helped in initiating the process of efficient and timely diagnosis which further helped them in classifying those affected by the coronavirus into four groups. For example, they have been able to develop a hand-held chest X-ray camera which can be used for scanning the chest of the patient in just three seconds. Furthermore, mobile apps were used for information sharing related to healthcare staff, volunteers, testing stations, point of purchase for available masks, etc. Robots using AI technologies were also manufactured and were being used by the authorities to provide information to the people on different ways of responses to this infectious virus.

6 Conclusions

There are many ways to tackle the contagious pandemic but the best one is social distancing or self-isolation, and the technologies related to artificial intelligence have contributed in facilitating it, for the control of this disease. The role of AI in combating this infection can be understood at various levels, i.e., from predicting the spread in the hotspots to assisting the prevention by facilitating social distancing, from guiding in discovering the treatment to planning the policies so that such type of pandemic can be avoided in the future. There are numerous examples which depict the contribution of AI in our daily lives but during this period of turmoil. AI-related tools and technologies have contributed much and the experts are working hard to device measures to further strengthen its contribution. There is an AI-based detector which act as a tool that issues an alert when anyone is less than the desired distance from a colleague at a workplace. Another AI company in USA unveiled a new feature in its interface for construction site workers, which was able to point out the indicators related to safety, productivity and quality, that include worker proximity and their use of personal protective equipment. Such examples along with many more have proved the potential use of AI in developing a solution for combating this infectious illness.

Social distancing, be it in the form of self-isolation, quarantine or at the workplace, is essential for the prevention of the spread of COVID-19 and is being facilitated by the tools and technologies related to AI.

References

1. Adams, R. L. (2017). 10 Powerful examples of artificial intelligence in use today. *Forbes,* Jan 10, 2017. www.forbes.com.
2. Chen, S. (2020). Taiwan sets example for world on how to fight Coronavirus. *ABC NEWS*, March 13, 2020. https://abcnews.go.com/Health/taiwan-sets-world-fight-coronavirus/story?id=69552462.
3. Ducharme, J. (2020). https://time.com/5791661/who-coronavirus-pandemic-declaration/.
4. Fong, S. J., Li, G., Dey, N., Crespo, R. G., & Herrera-Viedma, E. (2020). Finding an accurate early forecasting model from small dataset: A case of 2019-ncov novel coronavirus outbreak. *arXiv preprint* arXiv:2003.10776.
5. Fong, S. J., Li, G., Dey, N., Crespo, R. G., & Herrera-Viedma, E. (2020). Composite Monte Carlo decision making under high uncertainty of novel coronavirus epidemic using hybridized deep learning and fuzzy rule induction. *Applied Soft Computing*, 106282.
6. ITU News. (2020). COVID-19: How Korea is using innovative technology and AI to flatten the curve. *ITU News*, April @ 2020. www.News.itu.int/covid-19-how-korea-is-using-innovative-technology-andai-to-flatten-the-curve/.
7. Leo, K. (2020). Coronavirus: Covid-19 detecting apps face teething problems. *BBC NEWS*, April 8, 2020. www.bbc.com/news/amp/technology-52215290.
8. Santosh, K. C. (2020). AI-driven tools for coronavirus outbreak: Need of active learning and cross-population train/test models on multitudinal/multimodal data. *Journal of Medical Systems, 44*, 93. https://doi.org/10.1007/s10916-020-01562-1.
9. Sraders, A. (2019). What is artificial intelligence? Examples and news in 2019. *TheStreet*, January 3, 2019. www.Thestreet.com.
10. Webster's Dictionary. (2020). https://www.merriam-webster.com/dictionary/social%20distance#h1.

Post-COVID-19 and Business Analytics

Monomita Nandy and Suman Lodh

Abstract This paper highlights the way companies can apply artificial intelligence (AI) in the post-COVID-19 period. We show that how the AI can be advantageous to develop an inclusive model and apply to the businesses of various sizes. The recommendation can be beneficial for academic researchers to identify several ways to overcome the obstacles that companies may face in post-COVID-19 period. The paper also addresses few major global issues, which can assist the policy makers to consider developing a business model to bounce back the world economy after this crisis is over. Overall, this paper enhances the understanding of stakeholders of business about the importance of application of the AI in businesses in a volatile market in post-COVID-19 period.

Keywords Artificial intelligence · Crisis · COVID-19 · Artificial neural network · Coronavirus · Economic development

1 Introduction

The current COVID-19 outbreak, started in December 2019 in Wuhan city of China, brings an extraordinary crippling impact on the world economy. During this unprecedented socio-economic crisis for business, it is too early to recommend a business model for companies that can be useful when the world is out of the COVID-19 pandemic. Based on the existing literature on financial crisis or similar exogenous shocks, researchers have started predicting the effect of COVID-19 on world financial markets and direct or indirect impact on economic development (e.g. [1, 8]). After the failure of the Lehman Brothers in 2008, a strand of literature has evolved and

M. Nandy (✉)
Brunel Business School, Brunel University London, Kingston Lane, Uxbridge UB8 3PH, UK
e-mail: monomita.nandy@brunel.ac.uk

S. Lodh
Middlesex Business School, Middlesex University London, The Burroughs, Hendon, London NW4 4BT, UK
e-mail: s.lodh@mdx.ac.uk

© The Author(s), under exclusive license to Springer Nature Singapore Pte Ltd. 2020   83
A. Joshi et al. (eds.), *Intelligent Systems and Methods to Combat Covid-19*,
SpringerBriefs in Computational Intelligence,
https://doi.org/10.1007/978-981-15-6572-4_10

started discussing the 'Space Economy' that focuses on the application of advanced technologies such as the artificial intelligence (AI). Extant studies on the AI show the applicability and effectiveness of the AI in restructuring and reorganisation of economies and financial markets across the world (see [13, 14]). To initiate the economic development and reduction of inequality in allocation of resources for development of stakeholders, application of this technology receives an immense importance in academia and practice. Based on the above discussion, the objective of this paper is to identify the scope of application of the AI by companies in the post-COVID-19 crisis period as there is a lack of detailed studies on the impact of the use of the AI to overcome a pandemic shock similar to the one we are experiencing at the beginning of the year 2020. To the best of our knowledge, this original research is the first study to highlight the possibility of application of the AI by companies in the COVID-19 recovery phase.

2 Advantages of Using the AI After the End of COVID-19 Crisis

Companies can maximise the value of their concerns by minimising the operating cost. Porter [19] argues that companies apply their sustainable models to take competitive advantages over their peers. One of the main challenges faced by companies during the last decade is to deal with big data created by high information flow through the Internet. To address this challenge, companies start utilising the AI to improve the world economy [15]. Similar to big companies, small- and medium-size enterprises with the government interventions allow themselves to think in a creative manner. In addition, these companies introduce several disruptive changes in their businesses by applying the AI. The development of such infrastructure by big, medium and small companies positively impacts the rate of unemployment, GDP and inflation, to name a few, of many countries [17]. Moreover, an application of the super-intelligent system creates new scopes for business of various sizes and allows the transmission of required information within a few nanoseconds. As a result, the development of the economy becomes visible because companies, mostly in advanced countries, of all sizes can apply this sophisticated and efficient business model based on advance technology such as the AI. In fact, the analysis of big data allows the companies to reduce the percentage of error in their business model. Furthermore, the global coordination and participation has increased because of the application of these advanced technologies as knowledge and research and development (R&D) begin to transmit widely from one country to another.

Competition among peers in the same industry or between big and small businesses influences innovation to find a sustainable business model. The AI-based models allow companies to reach rural or underdeveloped areas by introducing user-friendly technologies in day-to-day life. For example, a digital-biological converter can make a number of copies of flu vaccines remotely in the absence of human to support the local health system [2]. Thus, various sectors such as health, transport, manufacturing and agriculture contribute to the development of the country-level economy, which in turn affects the world economy. During the financial crisis in 2008, the application of the AI by companies remains largely limited. However, recently, due to rapid advancement of technologies, companies are trying to apply a composite Monte Carlo decision-making process in the highly uncertain post-coronavirus period [5, 6]. In contrast, before applying the AI-based models to recover the economy from the current crisis, companies need to consider the unprecedented damage caused by the novel coronavirus which is not comparable with the previous financial crises, e.g. collapse of the Lehman Brothers.

3 Application of AI for Global Development in Post-COVID-19

One of the major global challenges for the past decades is to keep the global warming stay below 2 °C to reduce the risk of biodiversity. The rapid climate change is posing a high risk to the livelihoods of human being and to animal kingdom. A huge number of studies indicate that failure to conserve wildlife can create a threat to human being (https://www.eauc.org.uk/6998). In addition, the modern business activities are causing damage to environment, and this in turn can allow the harmful virus to find shelter in human being. Thus, the wildlife conservation needs to take care of a large database associated to business, which is difficult to obtain manually. In other words, companies need to identify the habitats to protect and then create wildlife corridors as these corridors have immense biological significance. Let us take the case of Montana and Idaho in the USA. The conservation scientists of wild animal are using the AI-assisted system to track and record the movements of wild animals. As a result, to reduce the risks associated with biodiversity, company can use the AI-embedded technologies and can continue to work on maintaining the climate change in the post-COVID-19 pandemic period.

The immense use of the AI can be observed in the healthcare sector, which is a big challenge for all countries around the world. During the recent pandemic, we observe the use of AI-driven tools and importance of active learning and cross-population test models [22]. For instance, robots can disinfect hospitals to support the health workers, 3D printers can manufacture the personal protective equipment (PPE) for health workers in hospitals and care homes, smartphone enabled-tracking system can identify the close contact of a person with another infected person, etc. are few to mention. Similar to the COVID-19 pandemic, we can also observe an application of the AI by healthcare business in the past decades. For example, the AI system of IBM Watson Health, in partnership with Barrow Neurological Institute, has been used to manage in analysis of many studies to conclude about the genes related to Amyotrophic Lateral Sclerosis (ALS) disease. In addition, remote treatment without risking the life of health carer is only possible by the application of advanced technology. Consequently, once we come out of the crisis, it is important for the companies to analyse a huge amount of information available from every affected country through their AI-based forecasting model. This can mitigate the risk of encountering the similar pandemic in the future.

In the recent days, we observe a huge investment in developed and developing countries by the public and private businesses for clean energy (Bloomberg NEF). In the post-COVID-19 era, the business can start utilizing the invested resources and generate more units of clean energy (or green energy) with the help of AI-based technology. For example, quantum computing can create plasma reaction in a nuclear fusion reactor which can reduce fuel-based energy and produce clean energy. Companies can also focus on assisting large businesses to find a technology-enhanced way of controlling the cost associated with the cooling system in the big data centre. Deep mind is one of the examples of cost-saving smarter energy used by big business, like Google.

The non-self-improving AI can create philosophical zombies (p-zombies), where we can observe a dead subjectivity. By combining the AI with the existing technologies, companies can address complicated problems through biological or artificial neural networks [4] or they can use the AI that do not self-improve even after interacting with the government structures. Industry can focus more on a short period for accurate early forecasting model using small dataset to check the suitability of an application of the AI [5, 6]. If businesses can get knowledge about how to reduce the cost of application of AI, how to merge the AI to time [3] and how to control various parameters of global issues by application of the AI [28]. As a result, the global control system can introduce a limited super-intelligence for the benefit of the society [7].

4 An Experiment on Application of the AI on Forecasting Cryptocurrency

Let us take a practical application of the AI on a real-time data. In this section, we show the use of artificial intelligence, especially an application of artificial neural network (ANN) in time-series forecasting. Similar to the function of human brains, the ANN is composed of a large number of highly interconnected processing elements. Currently, the application of neural network is considered as one of the most sophisticated methods for natural language processing and computer data visioning. For instance, in a study on bankruptcy prediction of banks and firms, Kumar and Ravi [11] find that ANN algorithm can outperform many single or hybrid classical forecasting techniques such as ARIMA and GARCH. In this brief experiment, we use a combination of well-known neural network algorithms such as long short-term memory (LSTM), time-lagged neural network (TLNN), feed-forward neural network (FNN) and seasonal artificial neural network (SANN) to forecast a sample (time-series) of

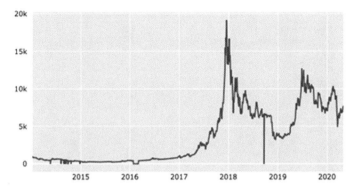

Fig. 1 Closing price of Bitcoin

cryptocurrency closing price[1] for the year 2014–2020 (till April 28, 2020). Figure 1 shows the time-series graph of a daily closing price data for bitcoin retrieved from Kraken.

To keep our analysis simple, we calculate the monthly average closing price in each year from the daily 2298 observations. We use 25% of this information as the test data and 75% data as the training data. In this training method, all the above-mentioned four models try to recognise the regularities and patterns in the input data, learn from historical data and then provide us generalised forecast values, based on the known previous information. Thus, the method is self-adaptive and non-linear in nature. So, it overcomes a priori assumptions of statistical distribution of the data. Based on the optimal parameters—such as root mean square errors (RMSE), our experiment suggests that LSTM model is a better method to forecast the bitcoin price movement. Our finding is reported in Fig. 2[2], and it indicates a downward trend of price of cryptocurrency since January of 2020. However, the model can be a complex one in practice if we consider transaction costs and other financial or environmental exogenous shocks such as economic lockdown due to COVID-19. Note that, our above-mentioned experiment is to show the applicability of ANN rather than drawing conclusion from the results for policy makers.

5 Challenges of Using the AI After the End of COVID-19 Crisis

The AI opens up a new chapter in the world economy. But, many studies, e.g. Roubini [20] and Stiglitz [25] raise serious negative implications of the application of AI in the World Economic Forum 2015 (WEF 2015). They mention that there is a need of huge investment of money and R&D to invest in the AI-embedded robots that can

---

[1] The data is obtained from www.cryptydatadownload.com.

[2] The other figures are reported in the Appendix.

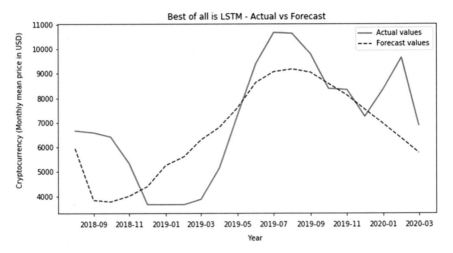

Fig. 2 forecast values of closing price

only be borne by large companies only. Thus, there is a limited opportunity to include both small and large businesses in the same model which may not be sustainable in the growing economy. Extant studies argue that a huge job loss can slow down the progress of the economy [12]. Popper [18] reports that the volatility can be higher in the economy when companies are able to use alternative digital money such as cryptocurrency. So, the lack of opportunities to small businesses can increase a higher gap in performance between public and private sectors or small and large companies. This may reduce the efficiency and accuracy in big data analysis and development of a business model applicable to all companies. The privilege of a group of companies with application of the AI may limit the development of the world economy. In addition, there can be a certain catastrophic AI risk. The challenges around the AI-safety or its alignment (see [21]) can be a huge concern for the companies, especially in the post-coronavirus crisis as there may be a lack of job force in practice.

As it is hard to be definite about the future uncertainties, companies can depend on forward looking taxonomy. One of the popular taxonomies, stated by Sotala and Yampolskiy [24], defines the dangerous impact of friendly AI [27]. For example, a bio-hacking of business can use AI to understand the published genomes, which might create a multi-pandemic [26] and such business model can create neural interfaces to affect the human brains adversely [10]. Thus, it still remains a puzzle as to what extent companies can apply the AI safely and effectively once the world economy gradually comes out of the COVID-19 pandemic.

6   Conclusion

In this forward-looking, constructive paper, we identify few challenges and yet major advantages that any business can take advantage in using the AI in the post-COVID-19 period. However, we acknowledge that immense challenges are waiting for us and the policy makers, around the world, should come together to solve these issues. One major challenge to the policy makers is to identify how to implement ethical practices in business to transmit data securely to get it analysed by AI-based technology for the benefit of the society. The local and international decision makers need to take responsibility to share their expertise to educate the mass about technology, which can reduce the risk of job loss. Moreover, by creating "Artificial Intelligence Marketing" [16], the restructuring of the world economic development is possible when the regulators allow the business to use the AI to enhance production-led profitability and to reduce the associated risk through innovative methods. Following the predictions of other studies, we expect that AI-led business can outperform all tasks of human as early as 2023 after the world economy manages to come out of COVID-19 pandemic (see [9, 23]). In a nutshell, the applications of the AI in the post-COVID-19 era can allow the individual and business communities to work together for the world development at a rapid rate by outweighing the negative aspect of using technology in society.

Appendix: Actual and Predicted Values from ANN Models

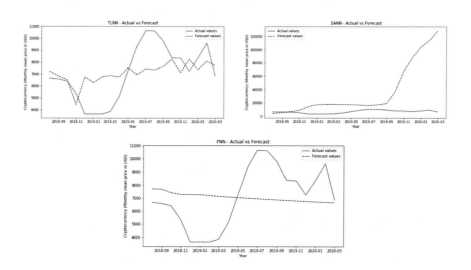

References

1. Bin, M., Cheung, P., Crisostomi, E., Ferrearo, P., Lhachemi, H., Murray-Smith, R., Myant, C., Parsini, T., Shorten, R., Stein, S., Stone, L. (2020). *On fast multi-shot Covid-19 interventions for post lock-down mitigation.* https://arxiv.org/pdf/2003.09930.
2. Boles, K.S., Kannan, K., Gill, J., et al. (2017). Digital-to-biological converter for on-demand production of biologics. *Nature Biotechnology, 35,* 672–675.
3. Bostrom, N. (2003). Astronomical waste: The opportunity cost of delayed technological development. *Utilitas, 15,* 308–314.
4. Christiano, P. (2016). *Prosaic AI alignment.* https://ai-alignment.com/prosaic-acontrol-b95964 4d79c2.
5. Fong, S. J., Li, G., Dey, N., Crespo, R. G., & Herrera-Viedma, E. (2020). Composite Monte Carlo decision making under high uncertainty of novel coronavirus epidemic using hybridized deep learning and fuzzy rule induction. *Applied Soft Computing,* 106282.
6. Fong, S. J., Li, G., Dey, N., Crespo, R. G., & Herrera-Viedma, E. (2020). *Finding an accurate early forecasting model from small dataset: A case of 2019-ncov novel coronavirus outbreak.* arXiv preprint arXiv:2003.10776.
7. Goertzel, B. (2012). Should humanity build a global ai nanny to delay the singularity until it's better understood? *Journal of Consciousness Studies, 19*(1–2), 96–111.
8. Goodell, J. W. (2020). COVID-19 and finance (2020) Agendas for future research. *Finance Research Letters* https://doi.org/10.1016/j.frl.2020.101512.
9. Grace, K., Salvatier, J., Dafoe, A., et al. (2017). *When will AI exceed human performance? Evidence from AI experts.* arXiv:1705.08807 [cs.AI].
10. Hines N (2016) Neural implants could let hackers hijack your brain. In: Inverse. https://www.inverse.com/article/19148-neural-implants-could-let-hackers-hijack-your-brain.
11. Kumar, P. R., & Ravi, V. (2007). Predictions in banks and firms via statistical and intelligent techniques—A review. *European Journal of Operational Research, 180*(1), 1–28.
12. Lalive, R. (2007). Unemployment benefits, unemployment duration, and postunemployment jobs: A regression discontinuity approach. *The American Economic Review, 97*(2), 108–112.
13. Lewis, Maureen. (2001). The economics of epidemics. *Georgetown Journal of International Affairs, 2,* 25.
14. Madhav, N., Oppenheim, B., Gallivan, M., Mulembakani, P., Rubin, E., & Wolfe, N. (2017). Pandemics: Risks, impacts, and mitigation. In: *Disease control priorities: Improving health and reducing poverty,* 3rd edn. The International Bank for Reconstruction and Development/The World Bank.
15. Manyika, J., Chui, M., Bughin, J., Dobbs, R., Bisson, P., & Marrs, A. (2013). *Disruptive technologies: Advances that will transform life, business, and the global economy* (Vol. 180). San Francisco, CA: McKinsey Global Institute.
16. Murray, S. H., & Keevil, A. A. (August 21, 2014). *System and method for interactive virtual banking,* Patent, No: US 20140236740 A1.
17. Öztürk, B., & Mrkaic, M. (2014). SMEs' access to finance in the Euro area: What helps or hampers? *IMF Working Paper,* WP/14/78. International Monetary Fund, European Department.
18. Popper, N. (29 April 2015). Can Bitcoin conquer Argentina? *New York Times Magazine.* http://www.nytimes.com/2015/05/03/magazine/howbitcoin-is-disrupting-argentinas-economy.html?smid=fbnytimes&smtyp=cur&bicmp=AD&bicmlukp=WT.mc_id&bicmst=140923272 2000&bicmet=1419773522000&_r=0.
19. Porter, M. E. (1985) *Competitive advantage: Creating and sustaining superior performance.* Free Press, New York, NY.
20. Roubini, N. (2014, December 08). *Rise of the machines: Downfall of the Economy.* http://www.roubinisedge.com/nouriel-unplugged/rise-of-themachines-downfall-of-the-economy.
21. Russell, S. (2017). *3 principles for creating safer AI.* https://www.youtube.com/watch?v=EBK-a94IFHY.

22. Santosh, K. C. (2020). AI-driven tools for coronavirus outbreak: Need of active learning and cross-population train/test models on multitudinal/multimodal data. *Journal of Medical Systems, 44,* 93. https://doi.org/10.1007/s10916-020-01562-1.
23. Shakirov, V. (2016). Review of state-of-the-arts in artificial intelligence with application to AI safety problem. ArXiv Prepr ArXiv160504232.
24. Sotala, K., & Yampolskiy, R. (2014). Responses to catastrophic AGI risk: A survey. *Physica Scripta, 90,* 018001.
25. Stiglitz, J. E. (2014, November). *Unemployment and innovation. Working Paper 20670* (Vol. 1050, p. 3). National Bureau of Economic Research. http://www.nber.org/papers/w20670.
26. Turchin, A., Green, B., Denkenberger, D. (2017). Multiple simultaneous pandemics as most dangerous global catastrophic risk connected with bioweapons and synthetic biology. Rev Health Secur.
27. Yudkowsky, E. (2003). *HUMOR: Friendly AI critical failure table.* http://www.sl4.org/archive/0310/7163.html.
28. Yudkowsky, E. (2008). *Artificial intelligence as a positive and negative factor in global risk, in global catastrophic risks.* Oxford: Oxford University Press.

Printed in the United States
By Bookmasters